HOW TO LOSE WEIGHT QUICKLY
BY
JAGDISH KRISHANLAL ARORA

techbagg@outlook.com

While every precaution has been taken in the preparation of this book, the publisher assumes no responsibility for errors or omissions, or for damages resulting from the use of the information contained herein.

HOW TO LOSE WEIGHT QUICKLY

First edition. January 6, 2024.

Written by Jagdish Krishanlal Arora.

Also by Jagdish Krishanlal Arora

Table of Contents

Also By Jagdish Arora

Also By Jagdish Arora

Introduction

A SUCCESSFUL WEIGHT loss is often achieved through a combination of healthy eating habits, regular physical activity, and lifestyle changes. You can make your own daily, weekly or monthly weight loss plans from this book. Here are some helpful guidelines:

Set Realistic Goals: Aim for a realistic and achievable weight loss goal. Losing 1-2 pounds per week is generally considered healthy and sustainable.

Balanced Diet: Focus on consuming a balanced diet that includes plenty of fruits, vegetables, lean proteins, whole grains, and healthy fats. Avoid or limit processed foods, sugary beverages, and high-calorie snacks.

Portion Control: Be mindful of portion sizes. Use smaller plates, bowls, and utensils to help control portions and avoid overeating.

Stay Hydrated: Drink plenty of water throughout the day. Sometimes thirst can be mistaken for hunger.

Regular Exercise: Incorporate regular physical activity into your routine. Aim for at least 150 minutes of moderate aerobic activity or 75 minutes of vigorous aerobic activity per week, along with strength training exercises at least two days a week.

Track Progress: Keep track of your food intake, exercise routine, and weight loss progress. This can help you stay accountable and make necessary adjustments.

Get Adequate Sleep: Aim for 7-9 hours of quality sleep per night. Poor sleep can disrupt hormones that regulate hunger and appetite.

Manage Stress: Find healthy ways to manage stress, as stress eating can contribute to weight gain. Practice relaxation techniques like yoga, meditation, or deep breathing.

Be Patient and Persistent: Weight loss takes time and consistency. Don't get discouraged by temporary setbacks. Stay focused on your long-term goals.

Seek Support: Consider joining a support group, working with a nutritionist or a personal trainer, or involving friends and family in your journey for encouragement and accountability.

Avoid Extreme Measures: Avoid crash diets or extreme measures for quick weight loss as they are often not sustainable and can be harmful to your health.

Focus on Health, Not Just Weight: Remember that weight is not the only indicator of good health. Aim for overall wellness by making healthy lifestyle choices rather than just focusing on the number on the scale.

Always consult with a healthcare professional or registered dietitian before starting any new diet or exercise program, especially if you have any underlying health conditions or concerns.

The human body is an intricate and remarkable entity, akin to a finely tuned machine with its own set of limitations and capabilities. Its appearance, weight, and overall functioning are intricately tied to the food we consume and our dietary habits. The body's transformation is a result of a complex interplay between various factors, including diet, lifestyle choices, genetics, and environmental influences. Understanding this dynamic relationship is crucial in comprehending how our bodies evolve and respond to our dietary habits.

The Body as a Machine:

The analogy of the body as a machine holds true when examining its functionalities and limitations. Just as a machine requires proper fuel and maintenance for optimal performance, the human body relies on nutrients obtained from food for sustenance, growth, and repair. Moreover, like a machine, the body operates within certain thresholds and capacities. Excessive strain, poor fuel, or neglect can lead to malfunction or inefficiency.

Food and Diet: Catalysts for Change

Our dietary habits serve as the primary driving force behind the body's appearance and weight. The food we consume serves as fuel for our bodies, providing essential nutrients, energy, and building blocks for cellular processes. Different dietary patterns elicit varied effects on the body's composition, metabolism, and overall health.

Nutritional Composition: The macronutrient and micronutrient content of our diets significantly influences our body's composition and weight. Balancing the intake of carbohydrates, proteins, fats, vitamins, and minerals plays a pivotal role in maintaining a healthy weight and promoting optimal bodily functions.

Caloric Balance: The body's weight and appearance are intricately tied to the balance between caloric intake and expenditure. Consuming more calories than the body expends leads to weight gain, while a caloric deficit results in weight loss. The quality and quantity of food consumed influence this delicate equilibrium.

Dietary Patterns: Various dietary approaches, such as low-carb, high-protein, plant-based, or Mediterranean diets, impact the body's composition differently. Each dietary pattern influences metabolism, satiety, and energy expenditure in unique ways, contributing to changes in body weight and appearance.

Impact of Habits: Beyond just food choices, habits like portion control, meal timing, hydration, and mindful eating significantly affect how the body processes food, stores fat, and utilizes energy.

Limits and Transformation:

While the body is adaptable and capable of transformation, it also has its limitations. Genetics, metabolic rate, age, and overall health status set boundaries on how much change is achievable within a certain timeframe. Rapid or extreme transformations often challenge the body's equilibrium and may lead to negative health consequences or rebound effects.

Healthy Transformations:

Optimal changes in body weight and appearance occur gradually and sustainably through a balanced approach that considers the body's limitations and capabilities. This involves making informed dietary choices, adopting an active lifestyle, and embracing realistic and achievable goals. Sustainable weight management involves a holistic approach encompassing nutrition, physical activity, stress management, and adequate rest.

Strategies for a Balanced Transformation:

Balanced Nutrition: Prioritize whole, nutrient-dense foods while moderating processed and high-calorie choices. Ensure a balance of macronutrients and micronutrients.

Portion Control: Monitor portion sizes to maintain a healthy caloric intake and prevent overconsumption.

Physical Activity: Incorporate regular exercise routines that align with personal fitness goals. Combining strength training, cardio, and flexibility exercises aids in body transformation.

Mindful Practices: Practice mindful eating, stay hydrated, manage stress, and prioritize adequate sleep to support overall health and well-being.

The body's appearance and weight are a reflection of the dynamic interplay between dietary habits, lifestyle choices, and physiological processes. Understanding the body's limitations and capabilities is fundamental to achieving sustainable and healthy transformations. By adopting a balanced approach to nutrition, exercise, and overall well-being, individuals can optimize their body's potential while respecting its innate mechanisms and limitations.

Chapter 1

THE PATH TO YOUR IDEAL Weight

Personalized Steps for Sustainable Change

Mindful Caloric Balance: Achieving weight loss involves the equation of consuming fewer calories than you burn. Merge increased physical activity with controlled calorie intake for effective weight management. Consult your dietitian for tailored advice on appropriate calorie levels and portion sizes that suit your body and goals.

Track Your Journey: Keep a personalized journal documenting not only your food intake but also your physical activities. Recording your progress can offer insights into habits and patterns, aiding in making informed decisions.

Weigh-In Ritual: Dedicate a specific day and time each week for a consistent weigh-in. Maintain similar conditions each time, such as clothing and scale used, to accurately monitor progress without unnecessary fluctuations.

Mealtime Consistency: Establish a routine for meal planning and timing. Regular, balanced meals, starting with a nutritious breakfast, can stabilize hunger levels and deter impulsive, unhealthy eating.

Designated Eating Spaces: Designate specific areas at home or work for meals. This practice helps to avoid mindless eating in other spaces and fosters mindful consumption.

Tech-Free Dining: Disconnect from screens during meals and snacks. Engaging in the eating experience without distractions promotes conscious eating habits and aids in recognizing satiety cues.

Savor and Pace: Practice mindful eating by slowing down and dedicating around 30 minutes for a meal. Allow 20 minutes before considering a second serving, as it takes time for the body to signal fullness.

Priority on Protein: Prioritize protein-rich foods at meals to induce a quicker feeling of fullness, helping manage portion sizes effectively.

Label Literacy: Educate yourself on food labels to control portion sizes and make informed choices about your nutrition intake.

Nutrient Focus: Emphasize a diet rich in fiber, found in fresh fruits, vegetables, and whole grains, while reducing intake of fat and sugar.

Mindful Eating Out: Limit reliance on restaurant and fast-food meals. Choose homemade options to have better control over ingredients and portions.

Environment Matters: Eliminate "problem foods" from your living and workspace—those tempting items that could lead to overindulgence when readily available.

Hydration Habits: Ensure adequate daily fluid intake of at least 8 cups (64 ounces) with a focus on calorie-free, caffeine-free beverages for optimal hydration.

Rest and Rejuvenate: Prioritize quality sleep of 7-9 hours each night to support overall well-being and healthy weight management.

Therefore, developing healthier eating habits and achieving weight loss involves a multifaceted approach that encompasses various strategies. Mindful eating stands as a pivotal practice, urging individuals to be attuned to their body's hunger signals and fostering a deeper connection with food. By embracing mindfulness during meals—eating slowly, savoring each bite, and eliminating distractions like screens—one gains a better understanding of satiety cues, leading to more controlled and satisfying eating experiences.

Central to a successful weight loss journey is the cultivation of a balanced diet. This involves prioritizing whole, nutrient-dense foods such as fruits, vegetables, lean proteins, whole grains, and healthy fats while minimizing the consumption of processed snacks, sugary treats, and beverages high in added sugars. Portion control plays an integral role; using smaller plates and bowls can help manage portions without feeling deprived, contributing to a healthier overall intake.

Establishing consistent meal times and avoiding skipping meals, especially breakfast, are vital components of a structured eating routine. Regular meals aid in preventing overeating due to extreme hunger and help maintain stable energy levels throughout the day. Staying hydrated by consuming adequate water is equally important, as it prevents dehydration and helps distinguish between thirst and hunger, reducing unnecessary snacking.

Pairing healthy eating habits with increased physical activity significantly contributes to achieving weight loss goals. Finding enjoyable ways to incorporate physical activity into daily routines—whether through cardiovascular exercises, strength training, or flexibility workouts—enhances overall fitness levels and supports weight management efforts.

Moreover, setting realistic weight loss goals—aiming for gradual and sustainable progress—is crucial. Creating a modest calorie deficit through a combination of diet and exercise helps achieve this. Keeping a food diary to track eating patterns and physical activities can provide valuable insights, allowing for adjustments as needed. Seeking support from professionals like registered dietitians, personal trainers, or joining support groups can offer guidance, motivation, and accountability on this journey toward improved health and well-being.

Ultimately, patience and persistence are key virtues in the pursuit of weight loss and healthier living. Celebrating small victories and remaining committed to long-term goals while embracing these strategies consistently will pave the way for lasting success and a healthier lifestyle.

Losing weight at a safe and sustainable rate is crucial for long-term success and overall health. The recommended rate of weight loss, typically 1kg (1lb to 2lbs) per week, ensures that changes are gradual and manageable. This rate allows the body to adapt to the changes without feeling overly restricted or deprived.

For most men, aiming to consume around 1,800 calories per day would support this gradual weight loss process. Similarly, for most women, a target of around 1,500 calories per day is recommended to achieve the desired weight loss within a healthy range. However, individual calorie needs can vary based on factors such as age, weight, height, activity level, and metabolism.

One effective way to determine a more personalized calorie target is by using a BMI (Body Mass Index) calculator. This tool takes into account specific individual metrics to calculate a more tailored daily calorie goal for weight loss. By inputting information such as height, weight, age, and activity level into the BMI calculator, individuals can get a more accurate estimation of the calories needed to reach their weight loss goals safely and sustainably.

It's essential to note that while calorie intake is a significant factor in weight loss, the quality of food matters just as much. Emphasizing nutrient-dense foods like fruits, vegetables, lean proteins, whole grains, and healthy fats within the set calorie limit ensures that the body receives essential nutrients for overall health while promoting weight loss.

Combining a balanced, calorie-controlled diet with regular physical activity is key to achieving and maintaining weight loss goals. Striking a balance between calorie intake, healthy food choices, and exercise will not only facilitate weight loss but also contribute to improved overall well-being. Always consult with a healthcare professional or a registered dietitian before making significant changes to your diet or exercise routine.

Increasing your fiber intake can significantly impact your overall health by promoting a well-functioning digestive system and potentially reducing cholesterol levels. In the UK, however, it's observed that the average daily intake of fiber among people is only around 18g, falling short of the recommended intake of at least 30g. To bridge this gap, it's crucial to incorporate more fiber-rich foods gradually into your diet.

The key to successfully increasing fiber consumption is to do it gradually to allow your body to adjust. Suddenly increasing fiber intake may lead to discomfort such as cramping and constipation. Therefore, it's essential to adopt a gradual approach by introducing fiber-rich foods slowly into your meals and snacks. This method gives your digestive system time to adapt to the increased fiber load, reducing the likelihood of digestive issues.

Additionally, adequate hydration is paramount when increasing fiber intake. As you consume more fiber, it's recommended to increase your water intake to ensure proper digestion and prevent discomfort. Aim to drink around 1.2 liters (approximately 4-5 cups) of water daily to support the movement of fiber through your digestive tract. Sufficient hydration helps soften stool and prevents constipation, ensuring a smoother transition as you enhance your fiber intake.

Including a variety of fiber-rich foods in your diet is a practical approach to meeting the recommended daily intake. Foods high in fiber include fruits like berries, apples, and oranges, as well as vegetables such as broccoli, carrots, and spinach. Additionally, whole grains like oats, brown rice, and whole wheat products, along with legumes like beans, lentils, and chickpeas, are excellent sources of fiber that can be incorporated into meals easily.

One way to increase fiber intake is by choosing whole grain options over refined ones. For instance, opt for whole grain bread instead of white bread or choose brown rice over white rice. Gradually swapping refined carbohydrates for whole grain alternatives not only increases fiber intake but also provides additional nutrients and contributes to better overall health.

Incorporating fruits and vegetables as snacks or side dishes is another effective method to boost fiber consumption. Try adding sliced fruits to your morning cereal or yogurt and including a serving of vegetables with your lunch and dinner. These small changes can significantly contribute to meeting your daily fiber goals.

Moreover, adding nuts and seeds to your diet is an easy way to increase fiber intake. Sprinkle chia seeds or flaxseeds on your cereal or yogurt, or snack on almonds, walnuts, or pumpkin seeds for an added fiber boost.

In conclusion, gradually incorporating fiber-rich foods into your diet is crucial to achieving the recommended daily intake of at least 30g. Doing so in a gradual manner helps prevent digestive discomfort such as cramping and constipation. Remember to stay adequately hydrated by drinking around 1.2 liters of water daily to support proper digestion and ensure a smooth transition as you increase your fiber intake. By including a variety of fiber-rich foods in your meals and snacks, such as fruits, vegetables, whole grains, legumes, nuts, and seeds, you can improve your overall health and promote a well-functioning digestive system.

Improving the fiber content in your morning meal can significantly affect your day, helping with satiety and possibly diminishing the craving for early in the day snacks. One straightforward yet compelling change is to trade out white bread for wholemeal or wholegrain assortments. Because these options contain more fiber, they help you feel fuller for longer and give you a more satisfying start to your day.

In addition, reexamining your cereal decision can essentially build your morning fiber admission. An excellent way to increase your fiber intake is to substitute wholegrain wheat cereals, unsweetened muesli, or porridge oats for sugary cereals. These choices offer a more prominent fiber content as well as give fundamental supplements without added sugars, adding to a more adjusted breakfast.

While making these trades, it's pivotal to be aware of the salt substance in bundled cereals. Checking the nourishing names guarantees that you're pursuing a healthy decision that lines up with your wellbeing objectives. Choosing low-sodium or unsweetened renditions of these high-fiber grains is the best way to deal with adjusting nourishing advantages while limiting the admission of pointless added substances.

Including foods high in fiber in your breakfast does not have to be bland or uninteresting. You can customize your morning dinner by adding new natural products like berries, bananas, or apples to your grain or porridge for an additional increase in fiber and normal pleasantness. On the other hand, including nuts, seeds, or dried natural products can likewise hoist the fiber content of your morning meal and give a brilliant crunch or chewy surface.

For those with an inclination for warm morning meals, oats or porridge is a flexible choice. Exploring different avenues regarding different fixings like nuts, seeds, nut spread, or a sprinkle of cinnamon adds flavor as well as improves the fiber content, making your morning meal both nutritious and delightful.

Whole grains in homemade breakfast options are an innovative way to get more fiber in your diet. For a nutrient-packed and fiber-rich start to your day, think about using whole grain flour to make whole grain pancakes, waffles, or breakfast bowls.

In addition, don't ignore the advantages of integrating protein-rich food varieties into your morning feast. Joining fiber with protein, for example, adding Greek yogurt or curds to your morning meal, can additionally add to satiety and give a balanced healthful profile.

Fundamentally, overhauling your morning meal to incorporate higher fiber choices like entire grains, unsweetened cereals, and new natural products or nuts is a down to earth method for upgrading your everyday fiber consumption. By making these basic yet significant changes to your morning schedule, you not just established a sound vibe for the afternoon yet in addition prepare for worked on generally speaking wellbeing and prosperity.

Chapter 2

WHEN IT COMES TO FOOD preparation, opting for low-fat cooking methods plays a pivotal role in crafting healthier meals. Embracing techniques such as baking, grilling, boiling, poaching, broiling, roasting, steaming, or microwaving without additional fat significantly reduces the overall fat content in dishes without compromising flavor.

Frying, known for its higher fat content due to oil absorption, is best avoided or limited in food preparation. Instead, using methods that require little to no added fat not only reduces the calorie count but also promotes heart-healthier cooking. For instance, placing meat on a rack while cooking allows excess fat to drain off, providing a leaner outcome.

Prior to cooking, removing skin from poultry and trimming visible fat from meat significantly reduces the fat content. This practice ensures that the resulting dish contains less saturated fat, promoting a healthier meal without compromising taste or texture.

Utilizing non-stick cookware or cooking sprays minimizes the need for additional fats or oils, offering a practical solution to reduce added fat content. This approach contributes to a lighter preparation method while preventing food from sticking to the cookware.

In recipes calling for eggs, substituting egg whites or egg substitutes for whole eggs is an effective strategy to lower cholesterol and fat content. These alternatives maintain the protein content while significantly reducing fat and calories in dishes.

Enhancing flavor without increasing fat content can be achieved through the use of spices, butter flavorings like Butter Buds®, lemon, or low-fat dressings. These alternatives add depth and zest to meals without relying on high-fat ingredients.

Moreover, when it comes to sauces and dressings, opting for low-fat alternatives helps reduce overall fat intake. Limiting the use of high-fat options like sour cream, regular salad dressings, full-fat gravy, and cream or cheese-based sauces such as Hollandaise or Alfredo sauce promotes a healthier dietary choice.

Replacing sugar with sugar substitutes in recipes tailored for baking or cooking reduces the calorie content significantly. These substitutes offer a sweet flavor without the added calories of sugar, making them an excellent choice for those looking to reduce sugar intake while still satisfying their sweet tooth.

Ultimately, adopting these healthier food preparation methods not only aids in reducing fat and calorie intake but also supports overall health. By incorporating these techniques into meal preparation, individuals can create flavorful, satisfying dishes without compromising on taste while prioritizing their well-being through mindful dietary choices.

Incorporating vegetables into your meals not only adds essential nutrients but also boosts your fiber intake. One effective strategy for lunch and dinner is to swap a portion of your usual meal components for more vegetables. Aim to have at least two portions of vegetables on your plate during dinner to increase your fiber consumption and promote overall health.

A simple yet impactful adjustment is to swap white rice and pasta for their wholemeal counterparts. This straightforward change can effectively double the amount of fiber in your meal. Wholemeal rice and pasta are rich in fiber, providing a more nutritious option that contributes to better digestion and prolonged satiety.

Another way to elevate the fiber content in your meals is by incorporating pulses such as beans, lentils, and peas. These legumes are not only cost-effective but also serve as low-fat sources of fiber, protein, vitamins, and minerals. Adding pulses to various dishes like soups, casseroles, rice, or pasta enhances both the nutritional value and fiber content. For instance, tossing beans or lentils into soups or stews creates a hearty and fiber-rich meal that's both nutritious and filling.

A versatile and popular way to include pulses in meals is by serving baked beans, preferably opting for reduced-salt and sugar varieties, on wholemeal toast. This simple meal offers a delightful combination of fiber, protein, and other essential nutrients, making it a wholesome choice for lunch or dinner.

Moreover, diversifying your vegetable choices can further enhance the nutritional profile of your meals. Experimenting with a variety of colorful vegetables not only adds visual appeal to your plate but also ensures a diverse intake of vitamins, minerals, and antioxidants. Incorporating leafy greens, cruciferous vegetables, bell peppers, tomatoes, carrots, and more introduces a spectrum of nutrients and flavors to your meals while boosting fiber content.

Crafting balanced and fiber-rich meals for lunch and dinner can also involve exploring whole grains beyond rice and pasta. Options like quinoa, bulgur, barley, or farro offer additional fiber and nutrients, contributing to a well-rounded meal.

By making these small but significant changes to your meal compositions, you elevate their nutritional value and promote a healthier lifestyle. Incorporating more vegetables, opting for wholemeal versions of grains, and integrating pulses into your meals not only enhances fiber intake but also ensures a well-rounded and satisfying dining experience that supports overall well-being.

Integrating fiber-rich snacks into your routine not only satiates hunger but also contributes to a healthier diet. When selecting snacks, opt for options that are abundant in fiber to promote better digestion and sustained energy levels between meals.

One of the simplest and most natural fiber-rich snacks is fruit, available in various forms like fresh, canned, or frozen. Choosing fruits like apples and pears and consuming their skin increases fiber intake significantly. The skin of these fruits contains valuable fiber and nutrients, making them a nutritious and convenient snack option.

Vegetable sticks such as carrots, celery, cucumber, or sugar snap peas offer low-calorie, fiber-packed snacks that satisfy cravings without compromising on health. These crunchy, low-calorie options provide not only fiber but also essential vitamins and minerals. They are an excellent choice to curb hunger pangs between meals.

Pairing vegetable sticks or whole grain crispbreads with reduced-fat hummus adds both flavor and fiber to your snack. Hummus, made primarily from chickpeas, is rich in fiber and protein, making it a nutritious dip. Combining it with vegetables or whole grain-based snacks enhances the overall fiber content of the snack while providing a satisfying and tasty option.

Air-popped, plain popcorn is a light and fiber-rich snack that can be made at home for a healthier alternative to store-bought versions. Homemade popcorn allows you to control the amount of added fat, sugar, or salt, ensuring a wholesome snack without compromising on flavor. Avoid adding sugar or butter to keep the snack low in calories and high in fiber.

For a more diverse range of fiber-rich snacks, consider mixing and matching these options. Creating fruit and vegetable medleys or combining different types of snacks allows for a wider variety of nutrients and flavors while still prioritizing fiber intake.

Furthermore, incorporating nuts and seeds into snack time provides additional fiber and healthy fats. Almonds, walnuts, chia seeds, or flaxseeds are excellent sources of fiber that can be easily added to yogurt, smoothies, or consumed as a standalone snack.

In conclusion, prioritizing fiber-rich snacks contributes to a balanced and nutritious diet. By choosing snacks like fruits, vegetable sticks, hummus, and air-popped popcorn, individuals can maintain satiety, manage cravings, and support overall health by ensuring adequate fiber intake throughout the day. Experimenting with various combinations and incorporating other fiber-rich options like nuts and seeds offers a diverse range of snacks that are both satisfying and beneficial for overall well-being.

Portion control is a crucial aspect of maintaining a healthy weight, regardless of how nutritious your diet might be. Despite consuming wholesome foods, excessive portions can lead to weight gain. Modern food portion sizes have significantly increased over the past few decades, resulting in unknowingly higher calorie intake—an issue known as portion distortion.

Restoring control over portion sizes can positively impact overall health. Here are six effective strategies to help manage portion sizes and avoid overeating:

Smaller Plates and Bowls: Opt for smaller dishware. Using smaller plates and bowls naturally limits portion sizes, allowing you to feel satisfied with a smaller amount of food. This psychological trick helps regulate serving sizes without feeling deprived.

Vegetable Emphasis: Aim to fill at least half of your plate with vegetables. Vegetables are low in calories but high in nutrients and fiber, promoting a feeling of fullness. By covering a significant portion of your plate with vegetables, there's less space for higher-calorie components, helping to balance your meal.

Mindful Eating: Slow down and savor your meals. Eating slowly gives your body time to signal to your brain that you're full. Rushing through meals often leads to overeating because your brain doesn't register fullness until it's too late.

Avoid Distractions: Eliminate distractions while eating, particularly the television. Eating in front of the TV can lead to mindless eating, where you're less aware of what and how much you're consuming. Focus on enjoying your meal without distractions to be more conscious of your food intake.

Portion Measurement: Consider using kitchen scales to measure ingredients before cooking. This practice ensures that you're following recommended serving sizes and helps avoid unintentionally large portions. Being mindful of serving sizes contributes to better portion control.

Be Mindful of Liquid Calories: Remember that beverages also contribute to overall calorie intake. Sugary drinks and high-calorie beverages can add up quickly. Opt for water or other low-calorie options to avoid excessive liquid calories.

Moreover, recalibrating our perception of portion sizes can be aided by referring to the Eatwell Guide, which provides guidance on balanced eating proportions. This visual representation helps in understanding the recommended portions of different food groups for a well-rounded and healthy diet.

In summary, being mindful of portion sizes is crucial for managing weight and promoting a healthy lifestyle. Implementing strategies such as using smaller plates, emphasizing vegetables, eating slowly, avoiding distractions, measuring portions, and being mindful of liquid calories can aid in regaining control over portion sizes and contribute to maintaining a balanced and nutritious diet.

Navigating restaurant dining or take-out while prioritizing a healthy diet involves adopting mindful strategies to make more conscious choices without compromising on flavor or enjoyment. When indulging in restaurant meals, managing portions and selecting healthier options can be pivotal for maintaining balanced eating habits.

To start, the selection of appetizers sets the tone for the meal. Opting to limit high-calorie starters like bread with butter or chips can prevent unnecessary calorie intake before the main course. Instead, considering a salad with a light dressing on the side or a broth-based soup not only serves as a healthier starter but also helps control overall calorie consumption.

When perusing the menu, it's wise to prioritize foods prepared using low-fat cooking methods. Grilled, steamed, or baked options tend to be healthier alternatives compared to fried dishes or meals laden with heavy sauces. This choice allows you to enjoy your meal without compromising on taste while aligning with your health goals.

Furthermore, being mindful of condiments is crucial. Requesting sauces, dressings, and gravies on the side gives you control over the amount you use, reducing excess calories and fat typically associated with these add-ons. By dipping into them sparingly or applying as needed, you can savor the flavors without overindulging.

Portion control techniques can also aid in managing intake. Consider the practice of setting aside a portion of your meal in a take-home container before commencing the meal. This preemptive measure helps prevent overeating by controlling portion sizes right from the start, ensuring you enjoy a reasonable serving.

Sharing an entrée with a dining companion is another effective strategy. Splitting a meal not only promotes portion control but also allows you to savor the dish while consuming a more appropriate serving size. It's a win-win, as you enjoy the meal while keeping portions in check.

For those who prefer to track their intake more closely, utilizing resources like pocket-sized calorie counter books can be beneficial. This tool offers valuable information on the nutritional content and calorie values of various foods, empowering informed decisions when dining out.

Ultimately, adopting a balanced approach to restaurant dining involves making conscious choices that prioritize health without compromising on taste or enjoyment. Implementing these mindful strategies allows for a more enjoyable dining experience while supporting your overall well-being and health goals.

Chapter 3

EMBRACING PHYSICAL activity as part of a healthy lifestyle is pivotal for overall well-being. The recommendation of aiming for 180 minutes of moderate-intensity exercise each week is a beneficial goal for maintaining fitness and health. If you've been less active recently, gradually increasing your activity levels is a prudent approach to prevent injury and allow your body to adapt to the changes.

Starting an exercise routine or ramping up physical activity after a period of inactivity requires a gradual and strategic approach. Begin by incorporating shorter bouts of exercise into your daily routine, such as taking brisk walks, cycling, or engaging in gentle yoga or stretching sessions. This initial phase helps condition your body for more strenuous activities over time.

Consider integrating various forms of physical activity that you enjoy. Whether it's dancing, swimming, hiking, or participating in team sports, finding activities that bring joy and fulfillment can make the journey toward achieving 180 minutes of exercise each week more enjoyable and sustainable.

It's essential to listen to your body and gradually progress without pushing too hard too soon.

Incrementally increasing the duration and intensity of your workouts over a few weeks allows your body to adapt to the increased demands, reducing the risk of injury or burnout.

Moreover, consistency is key. Strive for a routine that incorporates physical activity into your daily life. This can involve scheduling workouts at specific times, setting realistic goals, and creating a supportive environment conducive to maintaining an active lifestyle.

Remember, physical activity isn't solely about structured workouts. Incorporating movement into your daily life is equally important. Simple changes like taking the stairs instead of the elevator, walking or cycling for short errands, or incorporating short exercise breaks during long periods of sitting can significantly contribute to reaching your weekly activity goal.

While striving for 180 minutes of exercise per week is an excellent guideline, it's crucial to understand that any amount of physical activity offers health benefits. Even small steps toward increased movement and reduced sedentary behavior contribute positively to overall health.

Besides physical health, regular exercise offers numerous mental and emotional benefits. Engaging in physical activity can boost mood, reduce stress, improve sleep quality, and enhance overall well-being. This holistic approach to health emphasizes the importance of an active lifestyle beyond just physical fitness.

Consulting with a healthcare professional or a fitness expert can provide tailored guidance based on your individual needs, ensuring a safe and effective progression toward achieving the recommended 150 minutes of physical activity per week. They can help design a personalized plan that considers your current fitness level, health goals, and any underlying health conditions.

In summary, embarking on a journey toward regular physical activity is a positive step toward a healthier and more fulfilling life. By gradually increasing your activity levels and incorporating diverse and enjoyable forms of exercise into your routine, you not only meet recommended guidelines but also foster an enduring habit that promotes overall health and well-being.

Chapter 4

UNDERSTANDING FOOD groups and recommended portion sizes is crucial for maintaining a balanced and nutritious diet. Each food group offers distinct benefits, and knowing the appropriate serving sizes helps in creating well-rounded meals.

Meat and protein-rich foods are essential for growth and repair. Aim for 2-3 servings daily, where one serving equals 3 ounces of meat, poultry, or fish. Alternatively, 1½ cups of cooked beans, lentils, or split peas, ½ cup of tofu, or 2 eggs can be considered a serving. Choosing lean protein sources like poultry without skin, baked fish, egg whites, or meat substitutes can offer vital nutrients while reducing saturated fat intake.

Bread and starch-based foods provide energy and essential nutrients. Aim for 4-8 servings daily, where a serving equals ½ cup of rice, pasta, or cereal, 1 slice of bread, or ½ of a small bagel. Opting for whole-grain options like whole-grain bread, brown rice, whole-grain pasta, or whole grain crackers provides more fiber and nutrients compared to refined grains.

Fruits offer vitamins, minerals, and fiber necessary for overall health. Aim for 2-4 servings daily, where one serving equals 1 small piece of fruit,

½ cup of cut-up fruit, or ½ cup of fruit juice. Prioritize fresh fruits, frozen fruit without added sugar, or fruit canned in water or juice, as these options contain fewer added sugars and preservatives.

Choosing food options more frequently from the "choose more often" list ensures a healthier diet. Lean meats, whole grains, and fresh fruits offer more nutritional value and fewer unhealthy fats or sugars compared to options listed in the "choose less often or avoid" category. Limiting or avoiding foods like bacon, fried chicken, sweetened cereals, or high-fat crackers helps reduce intake of unhealthy fats, sugars, and processed ingredients.

By incorporating a variety of foods from the recommended list and being mindful of portion sizes, it's possible to create well-balanced meals that meet nutritional needs while supporting overall health. Moderation and variety play key roles in maintaining a healthy diet, ensuring an array of nutrients without excessive intake of less healthy options like fried foods, high-fat meats, and sugary snacks. Always consider individual dietary needs and preferences when making food choices to create a sustainable and enjoyable eating pattern.

Each food group offers distinct benefits, and knowing the appropriate serving sizes helps in creating well-rounded meals.

Vegetables play a crucial role in providing essential vitamins, minerals, and fiber. Aim for 3 or more servings daily, where one serving equals ½ cup. Opt for fresh, frozen, or canned vegetables prepared without added fat for maximum nutritional value. Additionally, incorporating broth-based vegetable soups is an excellent way to increase vegetable intake while keeping calorie counts low.

Dairy and milk products are vital for bone health and provide calcium and protein. Aim for 2-3 servings daily, where one serving equals 8 ounces of milk or yogurt, 1 ounce of cheese, or ¼ cup of cottage cheese. Choose nonfat or low-fat options like 1% milk, nonfat or low-fat cheese, nonfat or low-fat cottage cheese, and nonfat or low-fat yogurt to reduce saturated fat intake while still benefiting from essential nutrients.

Opting for foods more frequently from the "choose more often" list ensures a healthier diet. Fresh, frozen, or canned vegetables prepared without added fats, along with nonfat or low-fat dairy products, offer essential nutrients with fewer unhealthy fats or sugars compared to options listed in the "choose less often or avoid" category. Limiting or avoiding foods like creamed vegetable soups, fried vegetables, high-fat cheeses, and high-sugar dairy products helps maintain a balanced diet with fewer unhealthy additives.

Fats, while essential in moderation, should be used sparingly due to their higher calorie content. One serving of fats equals 1 teaspoon of butter or oil or 1 tablespoon of reduced-fat margarine or mayonnaise. It's essential to monitor intake of fats, opting for healthier sources like olive oil or reduced-fat spreads while limiting saturated fats found in butter, cream, and animal fats like bacon grease or lard.

By incorporating a variety of foods from the recommended list and being mindful of portion sizes, it's possible to create well-balanced meals that meet nutritional needs while supporting overall health. Moderation and variety play key roles in maintaining a healthy diet, ensuring an array of nutrients without excessive intake of less healthy options like fried foods, high-fat cheeses, and sugary dairy products. Always consider individual dietary needs and preferences when making food choices to create a sustainable and enjoyable eating pattern.

Understanding empty calorie foods—those high in fat and/or sugar but low in essential nutrients—is crucial for making informed dietary choices. Identifying these foods and their impact on overall health is instrumental in creating a balanced and nutritious eating pattern.

Empty calorie foods encompass a wide range of items, from sugary treats like candy, cake, cookies, and doughnuts to high-fat options like cream, cream cheese, and fried foods. These foods tend to offer minimal nutritional value while contributing significantly to calorie intake.

Alcoholic beverages like beer, wine, and liquor fall under this category due to their high-calorie content and lack of essential nutrients. Sweetened beverages such as sodas, fruit-flavored drinks, and contain added sugars and little nutritional benefit, contributing to empty calories and potential health issues.

Pastries, pies, croissants, and other baked goods often contain high levels of added sugars and unhealthy fats, making them contributors to empty calorie consumption. Similarly, creamy sauces like gravy, cream sauce, and tartar sauce contain significant amounts of fats and calories with minimal nutritional value.

Understanding the impact of empty calorie foods on health is essential for making healthier choices. Regular consumption of these items can contribute to weight gain, increased risk of chronic diseases like diabetes and heart disease, and a lack of essential nutrients vital for overall health.

While it's unrealistic and unnecessary to completely eliminate empty calorie foods, moderation is key. Reducing the intake of these items and replacing them with nutrient-dense alternatives is crucial for maintaining a balanced diet. For instance, replacing sugary beverages with water, herbal teas, or fresh fruit-infused water can significantly reduce empty calorie consumption.

Opting for healthier dessert alternatives like fresh fruit, yogurt with natural sweeteners, or homemade treats using healthier ingredients can satisfy sweet cravings while reducing empty calorie intake. Substituting fried foods with baked, grilled, or steamed options contributes to healthier eating patterns.

Reading food labels and being aware of added sugars, unhealthy fats, and high-calorie content in processed foods can help in making informed choices. It's essential to prioritize whole, nutrient-dense foods such as fruits, vegetables, lean proteins, whole grains, and healthy fats to ensure a well-balanced diet while minimizing empty calorie intake.

Incorporating mindful eating habits, such as being conscious of portion sizes, eating slowly, and enjoying treats in moderation, can aid in reducing the consumption of empty calorie foods without feeling deprived.

Overall, being mindful of the impact of empty calorie foods on overall health and making conscious choices to limit their intake while prioritizing nutrient-dense options is key to achieving and maintaining a healthy lifestyle. Balancing occasional indulgences with a predominantly wholesome diet supports overall well-being and long-term health goals.

Understanding and incorporating free foods—those with 20 calories or less per serving—can be a valuable component of a balanced diet. These foods offer minimal calories while providing flavor, variety, and versatility to meals and snacks without significantly impacting overall calorie intake.

Free foods encompass a variety of options that are low in calories but rich in taste and can complement meals in various ways. Broth, for instance, adds depth and flavor to soups and stews without contributing significant calories. Similarly, coffee, tea, and diet soda are refreshing beverages with minimal calories that can be enjoyed throughout the day.

Fat-free salad dressing and mayonnaise alternatives offer zest to salads and sandwiches without the calorie load of their regular counterparts. These substitutes, paired with lemon, lime, or vinegar, can enhance the taste of dishes while remaining low in calories.

Herbs and spices are excellent additions to meals as they provide flavor without added calories. Garlic, for instance, adds a robust taste to dishes while being a free food. Salsa, another versatile option, can be used as a dip or a condiment without adding significant calories.

Sugar-free gelatin, sugar-free syrup, and reduced-sugar or sugar-free jam or jelly offer sweet options without the added sugars commonly found in other sweeteners. Sugar substitutes are also free foods that can be used to sweeten beverages or foods without contributing calories.

Incorporating these free foods into a daily routine offers the opportunity to enhance the flavor and variety of meals while keeping calorie intake in check. However, it's important to be mindful of portion sizes, even with free foods, as excessive consumption may add up in calories over time.

Tips for managing portion sizes include visual cues such as comparing a 3 oz serving of meat to the size of a deck of cards or a serving of fresh fruit to the size of a tennis ball. Utilizing measuring cups for dry and liquid foods helps in understanding and controlling serving sizes more accurately.

Opting for smaller plates, bowls, and glasses can aid in managing portion sizes visually. Additionally, using a food scale for cooked meats, nuts, and dry foods ensures precision in measuring servings.

While free foods offer versatility and flavor without significant calorie contribution, it's crucial to maintain a balanced diet by incorporating a variety of nutrient-dense foods. Combining free foods with fruits, vegetables, lean proteins, whole grains, and healthy fats ensures a well-rounded and nutritious eating pattern.

In summary, incorporating free foods into a diet allows for culinary creativity and taste enhancement while keeping calorie intake in check. Being mindful of portion sizes and combining these foods with other nutrient-dense options supports overall health and a balanced diet.

Understanding serving sizes is crucial for maintaining a balanced and healthy diet. It helps in controlling portions and ensures that you consume appropriate amounts of various food groups to meet your nutritional needs without overindulging in calories or unhealthy substances. Here are helpful tips to comprehend and manage serving sizes effectively:

Meat, Poultry, or Fish: A standard 3 oz portion of meat, poultry, or fish is approximately the size of a "deck of cards." This visual cue makes it easier to estimate the appropriate serving size when preparing or consuming these protein sources.

Cheese: When it comes to cheese, 1 oz is equivalent to 4 playing dice, 1 slice of American cheese, or 1 mozzarella stick. Keeping these comparisons in mind assists in moderating cheese intake, which can be high in calories and fat.

Fresh Fruit: A single serving of fresh fruit is approximately the size of a tennis ball. It's a straightforward and portable measurement guide, aiding in controlling portions and ensuring adequate fruit intake.

Baked Potato: For baked potatoes, a 3 oz portion is about the size of a small computer mouse. This analogy assists in gauging appropriate serving sizes, especially with starchy foods like potatoes.

Use Measuring Cups: Utilizing measuring cups for both dry and liquid foods helps in understanding serving sizes, making it easier to regulate portions accurately and maintain a balanced diet.

Consider Smaller Plates, Bowls, and Glasses: Opting for smaller dishware can visually create the perception of a fuller plate, aiding in controlling serving sizes without feeling deprived.

Food Scale: Using a food scale helps measure cooked meats, nuts, and dry foods more accurately, enabling you to adhere to proper serving sizes more precisely.

Understanding food labels is equally essential in making informed choices about serving sizes and nutritional content:

Serving Size: The nutrition facts provided on food labels are typically for one serving. Pay attention to the serving size when evaluating nutritional information.

Servings per Container: It's crucial to note how many servings are in the entire package, as consuming multiple servings can significantly impact calorie intake.

% Daily Value: This value indicates how much of a particular nutrient one serving of the food contributes to a daily diet based on a 2,000-calorie intake. It helps in assessing the nutrient content of the food product.

Compare Food Labels: Look for foods that are high in dietary fiber, vitamins (like A and C), calcium, and iron while limiting those high in total fat, saturated fat, trans fat, cholesterol, and sodium.

Limit Certain Nutrients: For better health, limit total fat to 3 grams or less per serving, sugar to 5 grams or less per serving, and sugar in milk and yogurt products to 12 grams or less per serving. Choose starches with dietary fiber of 3 grams or more per serving.

By employing these serving size tips and understanding food labels, you can make more informed choices about your diet, ensuring proper nutrition while managing portion sizes effectively.

Chapter 5

DEVELOPING A PLAN FOR exercise and adhering to a specific daily calorie intake are crucial components of achieving health and fitness goals. To achieve success, it's essential to strategize and commit to these objectives, integrating them into daily routines. Here's a comprehensive guide to effectively plan exercise sessions and maintain a targeted calorie intake.

Crafting an Exercise Plan:

Setting Goals: Begin by outlining your fitness objectives, whether it's weight loss, muscle gain, improved endurance, or overall health enhancement. Establish specific, measurable, achievable, relevant, and time-bound (SMART) goals.

Choosing Exercise Activities: Select exercises that align with your goals and preferences. Whether it's cardio, strength training, yoga, or a combination, ensure it's something you enjoy to maintain consistency.

Schedule Exercise Sessions: Allocate specific times for workouts, ideally incorporating them into your daily routine. Writing down these scheduled sessions increases accountability and aids in following through.

Variety and Progression: Incorporate variety into workouts to avoid monotony and continuously challenge your body. Gradually increase intensity, duration, or frequency to progress and avoid plateaus.

Prepare for Obstacles: Identify potential barriers to exercise and plan strategies to overcome them. This might involve adjusting schedules, having alternative workout options, or seeking support from friends or a fitness community.

Managing Caloric Intake:

Determine Caloric Needs: Establishing an appropriate daily calorie goal is crucial. While a general guideline suggests 1,500kcal for women and 1,800kcal for men, these figures are approximate and may vary based on individual factors like age, metabolism, activity level, and specific health goals.

Tracking Calories: Use reliable tools or apps to track your daily calorie intake accurately. Being mindful of portion sizes, meal composition, and nutritional content helps in managing overall calorie intake effectively.

Meal Planning: Plan balanced meals that incorporate nutrient-dense foods like fruits, vegetables, lean proteins, whole grains, and healthy fats. Preparing meals ahead of time or having healthy snacks readily available can prevent impulsive, high-calorie choices.

Hydration: Ensure adequate water intake throughout the day. Sometimes, thirst can be mistaken for hunger, leading to unnecessary snacking and potential calorie surplus.

Seek Professional Guidance: Consider consulting a registered dietitian or nutritionist to tailor a calorie intake plan that aligns with your specific needs, ensuring a sustainable and healthy approach to managing weight and overall nutrition.

Integrating Both Plans:

Synchronization: Align your exercise schedule with your calorie intake plan. For instance, consume meals rich in carbohydrates and protein before workouts for energy and muscle recovery.

Consistency and Patience: Both exercising regularly and managing calorie intake require consistency and patience. Sustainable changes take time, and it's essential to stay committed to the process rather than seeking quick fixes.

Record Progress: Keep a log of both exercise sessions and daily food intake. This record can help identify patterns, track achievements, and pinpoint areas for improvement.

Adjustment and Flexibility: Be adaptable to changes. If certain exercises or calorie goals aren't working, be open to modifying them while staying focused on long-term health objectives.

Celebrate Milestones: Acknowledge and celebrate accomplishments along the way, whether they're small victories in sticking to your exercise routine or meeting specific dietary goals.

Remember, the ultimate goal is not just short-term weight loss but overall health and well-being. By creating a structured exercise plan and maintaining a balanced approach to calorie intake, you're not only fostering weight management but also cultivating a healthier lifestyle for the long term.

Engaging in regular physical activity while monitoring your calorie intake is a proven method for successful weight loss and maintenance. However, for many individuals, especially those less inclined to exercise regularly, restarting a fitness routine after a prolonged hiatus can feel daunting. It's natural to feel unsure about where to start and how to gradually integrate exercise into daily life.

Starting small is a prudent approach. Integrating simple activities into your daily routine can pave the way for a more active lifestyle. For instance, opting to walk instead of taking the bus for short distances or using stairs instead of elevators can increase daily physical activity levels gradually.

In addition to these lifestyle changes, consider allocating specific days in the week for structured exercise sessions. The target of 180 minutes of moderate activity per week is recommended for overall health benefits. Moderate activity should elevate your heart rate and cause a slight increase in breathing without making it difficult to hold a conversation.

Examples of moderate activities include brisk walking, cycling, or swimming. If these activities don't resonate with you, numerous exercise plans available on platforms like NHS Choices cater specifically to beginners and offer diverse options such as Couch to 5K, strength and flexibility routines, and quick home workouts.

Before starting any exercise regimen, proper planning is crucial. Consider factors like acquiring suitable footwear, scheduling workout days, and identifying the most convenient time slots for exercise. Preparing in advance significantly contributes to initiating and maintaining an exercise routine.

Moreover, choosing an activity you genuinely enjoy is vital for sustaining motivation. If you find pleasure in the exercise, it becomes easier to commit to it regularly.

Increased physical activity levels may stimulate hunger, which is normal as your body requires more energy after workouts. However, it's important to be cautious about post-exercise snacking habits. Opt for low-calorie yet filling foods such as fruits, low-fat yogurt, or reduced-fat hummus with whole-grain pita to replenish energy without consuming excessive calories that could impede weight loss progress.

Embarking on a fitness journey, especially after a period of inactivity, is a significant step toward better health. It's essential to remember that progress might take time, and consistency is key to achieving sustainable results.

Additionally, it's advisable to consult with a healthcare professional or a fitness expert before commencing any new exercise routine, especially if you have underlying health concerns or medical conditions.

As you progress, focus on the positive changes in your overall well-being and celebrate the small victories. Regular exercise not only aids in weight management but also contributes significantly to improved physical and mental health.

Chapter 6

HERE'S A COMPREHENSIVE guide with unique insights on incorporating physical activity seamlessly into your daily routine, providing ten simple yet effective strategies to increase activity levels and burn more calories throughout the day:

1. Walking Revolution:

Walking stands as one of the most accessible and beneficial exercises. Seek a walking buddy or join a local walking group to make this activity more enjoyable and encouraging. Embrace the outdoors while enhancing fitness by simply putting one foot in front of the other.

2. Stairway to Fitness:

Avoid elevators and escalators; instead, take the stairs whenever possible. It's an effortless way to infuse more physical movement into your routine. By opting for stairs, even for a few floors, you increase daily activity levels significantly.

3. Running Milestones with Couch to 5K:

Consider the Couch to 5K program, an acclaimed running plan designed to help individuals gradually build up their stamina and endurance over nine weeks, culminating in a 5km run. This beginner-friendly program offers a structured approach to developing a running routine.

4. Park Workouts:

Utilize local parks for exercise. Download the Strength and Flex podcast series, providing a guided workout plan over five weeks. These exercises can be performed outdoors, combining fresh air with fitness training.

5. Active Commuting:

Opt for active travel whenever possible by cycling or walking part, if not all, of your commute to work. Choosing to walk or cycle instead of taking public transport provides an opportunity to incorporate physical activity into your daily routine.

6. Park and Stride:

If driving to work is necessary, consider parking further away from your destination. Utilize this opportunity to engage in extra physical activity by walking the remainder of the distance.

7. Workplace Exercise:

Explore the possibility of incorporating exercise sessions into your workday. Utilize workplace gym facilities or take advantage of lunch breaks for a brisk walk, swim, or engage in activities like squash to boost your activity levels.

8. Family Fitness Time:

Promote family bonding while staying active. Spend quality time with your children by taking them swimming or engaging in outdoor activities at the park or in the garden. Encouraging your family to join in fosters a healthier lifestyle for everyone.

9. Green Therapy with Gardening:

Discover the fitness benefits of gardening, an activity that doubles as a great workout. Tending to your garden not only promotes physical movement but also offers a therapeutic and rewarding experience. Consider cultivating an allotment for both fitness and social interactions.

10. Consistency and Enjoyment:

Remember, the key to sustainable physical activity lies in consistency and enjoyment. Find activities that resonate with you personally to ensure long-term commitment. Whether it's walking, running, cycling, or engaging in recreational activities, choose what you genuinely enjoy.

By implementing these diverse strategies into your routine, you can effortlessly elevate your activity levels, burn more calories, and embrace a more active and healthier lifestyle without making drastic changes to your daily schedule.

Chapter 7

UNIQUE INSIGHTS ON gradually increasing physical activity levels and incorporating healthier breakfast ideas for a positive start to your day:

Gradual Increase in Physical Activity:

Incremental Progress:

If the target of 180 minutes of exercise per week seems daunting initially, don't be disheartened. Focus on consistency and gradual progress. Even small bouts of activity count toward your overall fitness goals.

Start Small, Grow Strong:

Remember, any exercise is better than none. Begin with manageable activities and steadily increase intensity and duration as you become more comfortable and confident.

Consistency Matters:

Consistent effort matters more than aiming for perfection. Strive to incorporate regular physical activity into your routine, gradually increasing time and intensity.

Tracking and Building Habits:

Keep track of your progress. Create a log or use apps to monitor your activities. Consistency helps in establishing a habit, making it easier to stick to your exercise routine over time.

Adapt and Overcome Barriers:

Identify and overcome barriers that hinder your exercise routine. Whether it's lack of time, motivation, or resources, find creative solutions to adapt and stay on track.

Healthier Breakfast Ideas:

Balanced Morning Fuel:

Breakfast kickstarts your day, providing essential energy. Opt for balanced meals that include protein, healthy fats, and complex carbohydrates for sustained energy release throughout the day.

Protein-Packed Choices:

Incorporate protein-rich foods like eggs, Greek yogurt, or nut butter into your breakfast. Protein helps with satiety and muscle repair and growth.

Whole Grain Goodness:

Choose whole grains like oats, quinoa, or whole-grain bread for sustained energy release. They're rich in fiber, vitamins, and minerals, aiding in digestion and providing essential nutrients.

Fruitful Beginnings:

Add a variety of fruits to your breakfast, whether as toppings for yogurt, mixed in oatmeal, or consumed whole. They offer essential vitamins, antioxidants, and natural sweetness.

Healthy Hydration:

Start your day with water or herbal tea. Staying hydrated is crucial for overall health and can help kickstart your metabolism in the morning.

Establishing a Routine:

Set Achievable Goals:

Define realistic exercise goals and breakfast habits. Gradually increase activity time and intensity while diversifying your breakfast choices.

Morning Rituals:

Create a morning routine that includes exercise. Whether it's a brisk walk, a short workout, or yoga, scheduling physical activity in the morning sets a positive tone for the day.

Preparation is Key:

Prepare breakfast ingredients in advance to streamline morning routines. Overnight oats, pre-cut fruits, or meal prepping protein-rich breakfast options can save time and encourage healthier choices.

Accountability and Support:

Consider involving a friend or family member in your fitness journey. Sharing goals and progress with someone can provide motivation and support.

Celebrate Progress:

Acknowledge and celebrate milestones. Every step, whether it's adding a few minutes to your exercise routine or consistently choosing healthier breakfast options, is a significant achievement.

By focusing on gradual progress in physical activity and embracing nutritious breakfast choices, you're not just fostering a healthier lifestyle but also setting the stage for sustained well-being and vitality. Remember, every positive choice counts towards a healthier and happier you.

Chapter 8

MOTIVATIONAL STRATEGIES to enhance exercise adherence and sustain enthusiasm:

Overcoming Initial Hurdles:

Beginning a new exercise routine often leads to muscle soreness and mental barriers. Embrace this initial challenge; it's a natural part of starting afresh. You're transitioning, and these discomforts will soon be a distant memory as you progress.

Top 10 Motivational Tips:

Realistic Expectations:

Remind yourself of the purpose behind your desire for increased activity—better health and weight management. Understand this as a vital element in your ongoing journey toward wellness.

Plan and Schedule:

Integrate exercise into your weekly agenda. By proactively scheduling workouts in advance, you set a commitment and make physical activity a consistent part of your routine. Preparing gym bags or workout attire the night before streamlines the process.

Acknowledge Achievements:

Reflect on your weekly progress. Reviewing your food and activity chart helps recognize and appreciate the strides you've already taken toward your fitness goals.

Share Your Journey:

Engage others by sharing your exercise plans and accomplishments. Vocalizing your goals adds a sense of accountability and encouragement to persist.

Buddy System:

Seek a workout partner, friend, or family member to join your exercise routine. Having someone to exercise with offers support, feedback, and makes workouts more enjoyable.

Music as Motivation:

Curate a playlist of energizing tunes that invigorate your workouts. Music can be a powerful motivator, boosting your mood and intensity during exercise.

Flexibility in Activities:

Explore different exercises or activities if you find your current regimen uninspiring. Experiment with varied workouts like swimming or gym classes to discover what resonates with you.

Conquer the Starting Line:

Recognize that the hardest part of exercise is often the initial push to start. Once you overcome this hurdle, the rest becomes more manageable.

Set Achievable Goals:

Establish attainable objectives—small milestones such as increasing daily steps or opting for stairs instead of the lift. Recording these accomplishments aids in tracking progress.

Incentivize Success:

Reward yourself with non-food incentives for reaching milestones along your fitness journey. Treat yourself for achieving goals, reinforcing positive behavior.

By incorporating these motivational strategies into your routine, you'll cultivate a mindset that sustains your exercise commitment. Embrace these tips as tools to overcome challenges and stay motivated on your journey toward a healthier, more active lifestyle.

Some comprehensive tips to increase physical activity and lead a more active lifestyle:

Consult with Your Doctor

Before starting any new exercise regimen, especially if you have any health concerns, it's essential to consult with your doctor. They can provide guidance based on your health status.

Start Gradually

Begin with moderate intensity activities and gradually progress towards the goal of engaging in physical activity for about 30-90 minutes most days of the week. Ease into the routine to avoid injury and fatigue.

Find Enjoyable Activities

Engage in activities you genuinely enjoy. This will help maintain motivation and make exercising more enjoyable. Spread out your physical activity throughout the day instead of doing it all at once.

Reward Yourself

Celebrate reaching your activity goals with positive reinforcement. Treat yourself to new sports equipment, spend time on hobbies, or indulge in relaxing activities like a long bath.

Prepare for Weather Conditions

Have a backup plan for bad weather. If it's not feasible to exercise outdoors, consider indoor alternatives such as walking in a shopping mall.

Comfortable Footwear

Wear comfortable and supportive shoes, especially for walking. Keep your sneakers near the door as a reminder to walk more often.

Exercise Before or After Work

Incorporate exercise into your daily routine. You can exercise before work or bring a change of clothes and head straight for exercise after work.

Schedule Exercise

Make exercise a priority by scheduling it on your calendar. Treat it as an important appointment that you must keep.

Integrate Activity Daily

Develop habits that promote more activity in your daily routine. For instance, take the stairs instead of the elevator, park farther away to walk more, or choose walking over driving for short distances.

Variety in Exercise

Avoid monotony by diversifying your physical activities. Listen to music or podcasts while exercising or involve a friend to make it more enjoyable and engaging.

Use a Pedometer

Track your steps with a fitness tracker. It can serve as a motivation tool and help you set and achieve step-based goals.

Following these tips can assist in gradually incorporating more physical activity into your daily life, ensuring a healthier and more active lifestyle over time. Always listen to your body and adjust your routine as needed to prevent any injury or strain.

Chapter 9

HEALTHIER SNACKING and 100-calorie snack ideas to keep you energized between meals:

Healthy Snacking Habits

Snacking between meals is normal, especially when your activity levels are up, and you're feeling the need for a boost. However, it's crucial to differentiate between genuine hunger and mindless grazing. Opting for healthier snack choices can help manage hunger and maintain energy levels without exceeding your daily calorie intake.

Importance of Smart Snacking

When it comes to snacking, quality matters. Choosing nutrient-dense snacks packed with essential vitamins, minerals, and a balance of macronutrients is key. These snacks can sustain your energy levels and curb cravings, preventing overindulgence during main meals. Healthy snacking also aids in stabilizing blood sugar levels, enhancing mood, and supporting overall well-being.

Mindful Snacking Practices

Mindfulness while snacking is fundamental. Listen to your body's hunger cues rather than consuming snacks out of habit or boredom. Stay attentive to portion sizes to avoid excessive calorie intake. Additionally, keep hydrated as thirst can sometimes masquerade as hunger.

100-Calorie Healthy Snack Ideas

Here are some 100-calorie snack options that can satiate your hunger and maintain your daily caloric balance:

Apple Slices with Peanut Butter: Enjoy half an apple (50 calories) paired with one tablespoon of peanut butter (50 calories) for a satisfying mix of crunch and creaminess.

Greek Yogurt with Berries: Relish a small cup of plain Greek yogurt (70 calories) topped with a handful of fresh berries (30 calories) for a protein-rich and antioxidant-packed snack.

Baby Carrots and Hummus: Munch on around 12 baby carrots (40 calories) dipped in two tablespoons of hummus (60 calories) for a satisfying crunch and protein boost.

Rice Cake with Cottage Cheese: Have a rice cake (35-50 calories) topped with a dollop of low-fat cottage cheese (50 calories) for a light and protein-packed snack.

Hard-Boiled Egg: Enjoy a single hard-boiled egg (70 calories) for a protein-rich, grab-and-go snack.

Almonds: Grab a small handful of almonds (around 10 nuts - 70-80 calories) for a nutrient-dense snack packed with healthy fats and protein.

Celery Sticks with Hummus: Dip five celery sticks (around 20 calories) into two tablespoons of hummus (60 calories) for a refreshing and low-calorie snack.

Air-Popped Popcorn: Snack on two cups of air-popped popcorn (70-80 calories) for a light and satisfying treat.

Healthy snacking plays a crucial role in maintaining energy levels and preventing overeating during main meals. By incorporating these 100-calorie snack ideas and adopting mindful snacking habits, you can curb cravings, manage hunger effectively, and stay on track with your calorie goals. Remember, snacking sensibly and choosing nutrient-dense options are essential for supporting your overall health and wellness journey.

Nourishing Breakfast Ideas

1. Muesli, Fruit, and Low-Fat Yoghurt

Begin your day with a no-added-sugar muesli, a high-fibre choice that provides sustained energy. Add fruit to elevate your intake of essential nutrients, contributing to your daily 5 A DAY target. Complement this with low-fat yoghurt, rich in calcium and protein.

No-added-sugar muesli (40g) = 141kcal

Low-fat yoghurt (125g) = 81kcal

Medium-size banana = 108kcal

Total Calories: 330kcal

2. Wholegrain Breakfast Cereal with Semi-Skimmed Milk

Opt for wholegrain breakfast cereals for a fibre-packed start. Choose fortified varieties for added vitamins and minerals that support overall health.

Two Weetabix = 117kcal

Semi-skimmed milk (200ml) = 103kcal

Total Calories: 220kcal

3. Boiled Egg with Wholemeal Toast and Reduced-Fat Spread

Eggs are a nutrient-rich protein source, offering essential minerals and vitamins. Pair a boiled egg with wholemeal bread, opting for reduced-fat spread to keep it light.

1 large egg = 78kcal

2 thin slices of wholemeal toast with reduced-fat spread = 206kcal

Total Calories: 284kcal

4. Grilled Mushrooms and Tomatoes on a Wholegrain Bagel

Grilled vegetables like mushrooms and tomatoes add a nutritious touch to your breakfast and contribute to your daily vegetable intake. Opt for a wholegrain bagel for sustained energy.

Wholegrain bagel = 260kcal

4 large mushrooms = 20kcal

1 large tomato = 33kcal

Total Calories: 313kcal

These breakfast options offer a balance of essential nutrients, including fibre, protein, vitamins, and minerals, setting a healthy tone for your day. Incorporating these quick and nutritious choices into your morning routine ensures a fulfilling and nourishing start, supporting your overall well-being.

Chapter 10

CREATING AN EFFECTIVE and healthy eating plan within the confines of the workplace is crucial, considering the substantial time spent there. Frequently, work demands, stress, and lack of time can undermine our dietary goals, leading to poor eating habits. However, with strategic planning, it's possible to leverage snacks and lunchtime for maintaining a balanced diet, sustaining energy levels, and saving money.

Implementing these 10 tips can significantly improve your workplace eating habits:

1. Prioritize Breakfast

Kickstart your day with a nutritious breakfast to prevent mid-morning hunger. If you're not inclined to eat at home, having breakfast at work is an excellent alternative to keep you fueled until lunchtime.

2. Bring Your Own Food

Prepare home-cooked meals to bring to work. These meals are typically lower in calories and fat compared to high-street alternatives. Leftovers from dinner can also serve as a convenient and cost-effective lunch option.

3. Hydrate with Water

Drinking adequate water throughout the day can help stave off hunger. Aim for about six to eight glasses (1.2 liters) of fluid daily to stay hydrated and potentially reduce cravings.

4. Plan Healthier Snacks

Keep healthy snack options at hand, such as fruits, veggies (like carrot sticks paired with reduced-fat hummus), or homemade popcorn without added fats, sugars, or salt, to combat hunger between meals.

5. Choose Whole Grains

Opt for wholegrain bread for sandwiches as it tends to be more filling than white bread, keeping you satisfied for longer periods. Consider wholemeal pitta bread or bagels as alternatives to standard white loaves.

6. Opt for Lower-Fat Options

Reduce the fat content in your meals by swapping regular mayonnaise for lower-fat alternatives, such as reduced-fat mayo, hummus, tzatziki, or tomato salsa.

7. Boost Your Fruit and Veg Intake

Snack time is an excellent opportunity to increase your fruit and vegetable consumption. Each portion should amount to about 80g to contribute to your daily 5 A DAY goal.

8. Substitute High-Fat Snacks

Choose healthier alternatives to high-fat snacks. Opt for oven-baked crisps or plain rice cakes instead of regular crisps to reduce your fat intake during lunch.

9. Select Lean Protein Sources

When crafting your sandwiches, lean towards turkey, chicken, tuna, salmon, or hard-boiled eggs instead of fatty fillings like sausages or bacon. However, practice moderation with mayo.

10. Prepare Vegetable-Based Soups

Create lower-calorie, vegetable-based soups that serve as a satisfying and nutritious addition to your lunch. Make a batch during the weekend to enjoy throughout the week.

Implementing these strategies can transform your workplace eating habits, aiding in maintaining a healthier diet, improving energy levels, and supporting your overall well-being during work hours.

Chapter 11

EXERCISES

Incorporating a home workout regimen is a fantastic way to maintain physical fitness and stay active. The 15 Weighted Couch Squats are a perfect example of how everyday items, like a backpack, can be repurposed for exercise. This exercise not only targets the lower body muscles but also challenges the core. The action of standing from a seated position emphasizes the quads, hamstrings, and glutes, providing an effective lower body workout. To take it up a notch, turning it into a jump can intensify the movement, providing an additional cardiovascular challenge.

The 45 seconds of Mountain Climbers followed by Pushups form a dynamic exercise combo that incorporates both strength and cardio. This exercise sequence engages the core, arms, shoulders, and lower body. Mountain Climbers elevate the heart rate and engage the abdominal muscles, while the subsequent Pushups further strengthen the upper body and core, making it a comprehensive and efficient workout.

Including Overhead Presses with weighted objects helps target the deltoid muscles of the shoulders, strengthening the arms and upper body. It's an effective exercise for improving shoulder stability and overall upper body strength. The football goal post position ensures the correct form, while the overhead movement provides a thorough shoulder workout.

Bent Over Rows engage the back muscles, specifically targeting the lats, rhomboids, and biceps. This exercise is crucial for developing upper body strength and stability. The bent-over position activates the core muscles while ensuring proper form to effectively strengthen the back muscles.

The Full Body Crunches are a fantastic addition for targeting the abdominal muscles. This exercise not only engages the core but also works the entire body. The movement requires coordination between the upper and lower body, making it an excellent exercise for building core strength and stability.

Implementing these exercises into a workout routine can help develop overall strength, improve cardiovascular fitness, and increase muscular endurance. By targeting various muscle groups, these exercises create a well-rounded and effective home workout routine. They can be adapted for different fitness levels by adjusting the weight, repetitions, or intensity, making them suitable for beginners to more experienced individuals seeking a challenging workout. Additionally, performing these exercises in a circuit format can elevate heart rate, creating a fantastic full-body workout. Always ensure proper form and technique to prevent injury and maximize the benefits of each exercise.

Hip Thrusts:

Hip thrusts primarily target the glutes, hamstrings, and lower back muscles. Here's how to perform them:

Start by sitting on the floor with your upper back against a bench or couch and your feet flat on the ground, hip-width apart.

Roll a barbell over your hips or place a weight plate on your pelvis for added resistance.

Engage your core and drive your hips upward by pushing through your heels, squeezing your glutes at the top.

Lower your hips back down toward the ground without fully resting your bottom on the floor and repeat.

Bear Crawl Burpees:

This exercise combines elements of a bear crawl and a burpee to engage multiple muscle groups while enhancing cardiovascular fitness. Here are the steps:

Begin in a standing position.

Bend down and walk your hands out to assume a plank or push-up position.

Perform a push-up.

Walk your hands back toward your feet, returning to a crouched position.

Explosively jump up with your arms extended overhead.

Shoulder Taps:

Shoulder taps engage the core, arms, and shoulders while stabilizing the body. Here's how to execute them:

Start in a push-up position with your hands directly under your shoulders.

Keeping your hips stable and parallel to the ground, lift one hand and touch the opposite shoulder.

Return the hand to the starting position and repeat with the opposite hand.

Supermans:

Supermans target the lower back, glutes, and hamstrings to strengthen the posterior chain. Here's the technique:

Lie face down on a mat or the floor, arms extended in front of you.

Simultaneously lift your arms, chest, and legs off the ground while contracting your lower back and glutes.

Hold for a brief moment, then slowly lower back down to the starting position.

Leg Lowers:

Leg lowers focus on the lower abdominal muscles. Here are the steps to perform them correctly:

Lie on your back with your legs extended toward the ceiling, forming a 90-degree angle with your hips and knees.

Keeping your lower back pressed into the floor, slowly lower your legs toward the ground.

Stop when your legs are a few inches above the floor, then lift them back up to the starting position using your core muscles.

These exercises are effective for targeting various muscle groups and improving overall strength and stability. Consistently incorporating them into your workout routine can lead to improved muscular endurance, strength, and core stability.

Engaging in a comprehensive home workout doesn't always require complex gym equipment. The Sprinter Pulls serve as an excellent example of a dynamic lower body exercise that mimics the action of running. By starting in a lunge position and bringing the back foot forward while swinging the arms to simulate a running motion, this exercise targets the legs, glutes, and core. Executing eight repetitions per leg ensures a balanced workout and engages major muscle groups effectively.

The Lower Ab "U's" focus on targeting the lower abdominal muscles. By lying on your back with hands supporting on the couch, this exercise involves moving the legs back and forth, forming a "U" shape while ensuring the back remains flat against the floor. This movement engages the lower abs and helps strengthen the core, aiding in overall stability and balance.

Incorporating Romanian Deadlifts into a workout routine can significantly benefit the posterior chain. By standing and holding weighted objects in front of the thighs, this exercise involves hinging at the hips while maintaining relatively straight legs. The primary focus is on lowering the weights down the legs until a stretch is felt, engaging the hamstrings and glutes. The controlled movement back up to the starting position helps in building strength and stability in the lower body.

The Tricep Pushups are an effective upper body exercise focusing on the triceps, chest, and shoulders. Executing the pushups with elbows angled towards the back of the room ensures optimal tricep engagement. For modification, knee tricep pushups can be performed, allowing individuals to gradually build strength in their upper body.

Completing the workout with Three-Legged Dog Swings adds a dynamic element by transitioning from

Downward Dog to a three-legged dog position. Raising one leg towards the ceiling engages the core and stabilizing muscles, while the subsequent forward motion towards the shoulders challenges balance and coordination. This exercise sequence provides a full-body workout, targeting multiple muscle groups effectively.

Incorporating these exercises into a workout routine helps individuals strengthen various muscle groups and enhance overall fitness levels. By combining lower body, core, and upper body exercises, this routine offers a holistic approach to fitness. The exercises can be adjusted based on fitness levels, allowing beginners to gradually progress and advanced individuals to intensify the routine by increasing repetitions or adding resistance. Always prioritize proper form and technique to maximize the effectiveness of each exercise and prevent injuries.

Chapter 12

STRETCHING AND COOLING down after a run or workout is a vital part of any fitness routine. It helps the body gradually transition from the intense physical activity to a state of relaxation, aids in reducing muscle tension, improves flexibility, and minimizes soreness or potential injuries. Allocating around five minutes for post-workout stretching is essential to reap these benefits and optimize recovery.

Begin by focusing on the major muscle groups that were engaged during your workout. Start with the legs, particularly the quadriceps, hamstrings, calves, and hip flexors. A standing quadriceps stretch is a simple yet effective way to start. Standing tall, grab your ankle behind you and gently pull it toward your glutes, feeling the stretch in the front of the thigh. Hold each stretch for about 15-30 seconds, avoiding bouncing movements, which could lead to muscle strain.

Transition into a hamstring stretch by extending one leg out and bending at the waist to reach towards your toes. Maintain a straight back and avoid locking your knees. Hold this stretch for 15-30 seconds, feeling the tension in the back of your thighs. Repeat the same stretch for the other leg.

Moving on to the calf muscles, find a wall or a sturdy structure to perform a calf stretch. Place one foot behind you with the heel on the ground and lean forward, feeling the stretch in your calf. Hold for 15-30 seconds and then switch to stretch the other calf.

The hip flexors can be targeted with a lunge stretch. Take a step forward into a lunge position, ensuring your front knee is at a 90-degree angle. Keep your back straight and gently lower your hips forward, feeling the stretch in the front of the back leg's hip. Hold for 15-30 seconds and then switch to stretch the opposite side.

Transitioning to the upper body, focus on the shoulders, chest, and arms. A standing shoulder stretch involves bringing one arm across your body and using the opposite arm to gently press it closer to your chest, feeling the stretch in the shoulder and upper back. Hold for 15-30 seconds on each side.

Next, stretch your chest muscles by clasping your hands behind your back and gently lifting your arms while squeezing your shoulder blades together. Hold for 15-30 seconds, feeling the stretch across your chest and shoulders.

Finish with an overhead triceps stretch. Raise one arm overhead, bend it at the elbow, and gently grasp the elbow with your opposite hand. Gently pull the elbow towards the center of your head, feeling the stretch along the back of your arm. Hold for 15-30 seconds and repeat on the other side.

After completing the stretches, allow yourself a few minutes for a gradual cool-down. This could involve walking at a slower pace or practicing relaxed breathing exercises. Hydrating with water post-exercise is also crucial to replenish lost fluids.

Remember that stretching should be comfortable and pain-free. Never force a stretch beyond your comfort level, and avoid bouncing or jerking movements that could lead to injury. Consistency is key - performing these stretches regularly after workouts will contribute to improved flexibility, reduced muscle tension, and better overall recovery.

Chapter 13

UNDERSTANDING WHY WEIGHT loss efforts might plateau despite maintaining a strict eating regime is a common concern for many individuals. Often, unnoticed or overlooked factors such as beverage choices can play a significant role in impeding weight loss progress. It's time to delve deeper into how seemingly innocent beverages like lattes, flavored water, or evening drinks might impact weight loss goals.

The Latte Factor: Starting your day with a regular latte might seem harmless, but these caffeinated delights can carry more calories and sugar than expected. A typical latte can pack added sugar, whole milk, and even syrup, which contribute extra calories that might counteract your dieting efforts. Opting for alternatives like black coffee or unsweetened plant-based milk options can make a difference in reducing unnecessary calorie intake.

Flavored Water Dilemma: While flavored water might appear to be a healthy choice, some commercial varieties contain added sugars or artificial sweeteners that sneakily contribute to your calorie count. Checking the labels for hidden sugars and opting for homemade infused water with fresh fruits or herbs can provide the flavor without the unwanted additives.

Evening Tipple Trouble: Unwinding with an alcoholic drink in the evening is a common relaxation ritual, but alcoholic beverages can be high in calories and often lack nutritional value. The empty calories from alcoholic drinks can hinder weight loss progress. Choosing lower-calorie options, consuming in moderation, or alternating alcoholic drinks with water or soda water can be healthier choices.

Sugary Sodas and Juices: Another culprit in weight management might be sugary sodas or fruit juices. Often, these beverages are packed with hidden sugars that quickly add up in calories. Switching to water, herbal teas, or natural fruit-infused water can help reduce sugar intake without compromising taste.

Energy and Sports Drinks: Although marketed as replenishing energy, many sports drinks or energy beverages contain high levels of added sugars or artificial additives. Consideration should be given to their calorie content and whether the workout intensity justifies their consumption. Water and natural electrolyte sources like coconut water can be healthier options for hydration.

Mindful Hydration: Water, often overlooked, remains the best hydrating option with no calories or sugars. Staying well-hydrated is essential for overall health and can also aid in weight loss by promoting feelings of fullness and preventing overeating.

Portion Control and Moderation: Even seemingly harmless beverages can disrupt weight loss goals when consumed in large quantities. Being mindful of portion sizes and moderating the intake of these beverages can significantly impact calorie consumption and help maintain a calorie deficit for weight loss.

In summary, when aiming for weight loss, it's crucial to consider not only the foods but also the beverages consumed. Awareness of the hidden calories and sugars in seemingly innocent beverages is key to breaking through weight loss plateaus and achieving your desired health goals. Making informed and healthier beverage choices can contribute significantly to successful weight management.

Coping with Food Cravings

Our resolve often faces a rigorous test in the face of food cravings, regardless of our noble intentions. Understanding and managing these urges can significantly impact our willpower. Here are effective strategies to tackle and mitigate food cravings:

Uncover the Root Cause

Debate surrounds the origins of cravings, often stemming from emotional triggers like stress, boredom, habit, or insecurity. Identifying these underlying factors can aid in managing and eventually overcoming the cravings.

Stay Satiated

Combat intensified cravings by avoiding hunger pangs. Maintain stable energy levels with wholesome, high-fiber snacks to curb the desire for unhealthy indulgences.

Hydrate Wisely

Sipping water can alleviate cravings for some individuals. Its filling effect might deceive the body into a sense of fullness. Alternatively, opt for hot beverages as a substitute.

Engage in Diversions

Shift your focus away from cravings by immersing yourself in activities. A leisurely walk, a relaxing bath, a chat with a friend, or listening to music can effectively distract your mind.

Gum Chewing Technique

Chewing sugar-free gum has been known to suppress appetite. However, exercise caution as excessive consumption, surpassing 20 sticks a day, might lead to adverse effects.

Freshen Up

Utilize toothpaste to brush your teeth thoroughly. The minty sensation often helps dispel cravings, leaving a clean and refreshed palate.

Eliminate Temptation

Resist the urge for unhealthy choices by limiting their accessibility. Avoid purchasing these items, reducing the likelihood of succumbing to the cravings.

Time-Bound Strategy

Acknowledge that cravings are transient. Challenge yourself by imposing a 30-minute delay and engage in diversions during this period. Often, the desire fades away once the designated time elapses.

Controlled Indulgence

Should the craving persist, consider giving in sensibly. Opt for a small portion and compensate by adjusting your calorie intake later to maintain your overall health goals.

By employing these proactive techniques, one can successfully navigate and mitigate the impact of food cravings on their well-being, fostering healthier eating habits and bolstering willpower in the face of temptation.

Alcohol, often overlooked for its caloric content, surprisingly packs a caloric punch akin to indulgent treats. Despite conscious efforts to monitor food intake, many disregard the significant calories present in alcoholic beverages. This negligence can lead to unwelcome weight gain and hinder progress towards a healthier lifestyle.

Consider these eye-opening comparisons: a standard glass of wine mirrors the caloric content of a small chocolate bar, while a pint of lager rivals a packet of crisps in its calorie count. Unfortunately, this lack of awareness leads to a casual approach toward alcohol consumption, unlike the careful consideration given to high-calorie food choices.

Two pints of beer equate to the calorie intake of a full glass of single cream, an association often overlooked amid social drinking sessions. Such obliviousness contributes to the easily underestimated impact of excessive alcohol intake on weight gain.

Visualizing the calorie intake, two large glasses of white wine, amounting to 360 kcal, can constitute almost one-fifth of a woman's daily calorie allowance. The scale of consumption becomes glaringly apparent when a beer enthusiast imbibing just five pints weekly accrues a staggering 44,200 kcal over a year, the equivalent of devouring 221 doughnuts.

Alcohol itself contains a significant calorie load - seven calories per gram, almost akin to the caloric density of fat. Moreover, additional calories are often overlooked in mixer drinks. Furthermore, many augment their liquid calorie count by pairing drinks with high-calorie snacks like crisps, nuts, or pork scratchings, culminating in added weight concerns. Subsequent hangover-induced cravings often lead to a morning-after indulgence, adding an extra 450 kcal.

To counterbalance potential weight gain, consider implementing the following tips:

Adhere to Recommended Limits:

Men: Limit alcohol intake to 3-4 units daily.

Women: Restrict consumption to 2-3 units daily.

Alternate with Non-Alcoholic Options:

Hydrate by alternating alcoholic drinks with diet soft drinks or water.

Opt for Lower ABV Alternatives:

Choose beverages with lower alcohol content and fewer calories.

Mindful Eating:

Avoid drinking on an empty stomach and opt for lighter snacks if necessary.

Monitor Consumption:

Be mindful of drinking in rounds, as it often leads to unintended overconsumption.

Seek Support:

Consider reducing intake with a friend for added support and accountability.

Preemptive Measures:

Consume a healthy meal before drinking to curb unhealthy cravings.

Avoid Binge Drinking:

Drinking large quantities in a short period can severely impact health.

The comparison of various alcoholic drinks to common snacks illustrates the hidden caloric load, providing a clear perspective on the impact of alcohol on daily caloric intake.

Moreover, practical drink swaps can significantly reduce calorie consumption without compromising social enjoyment. Making informed choices regarding alcoholic beverages is essential when aiming for weight loss, complementing efforts toward a healthier lifestyle.

Beyond alcohol, non-alcoholic drinks can also contribute significantly to calorie intake, emphasizing the importance of vigilance and informed choices when considering all beverages in weight management strategies. Evaluating drink choices, being mindful of intake, and making informed swaps are pivotal steps toward achieving weight management goals.

Chapter 14

WEIGHT TRAINING OFTEN gets sidelined in many fitness routines aimed at burning fat. This omission, however, is a grave mistake. Weight training plays a pivotal role in preserving and fortifying our muscle mass, which is essential during periods of dieting. Failure to incorporate weight training during a dieting phase can result in the body utilizing muscle as an energy source, thereby sabotaging one's weight loss efforts. This scenario proves detrimental as muscle demands a substantial number of calories for maintenance. In simpler terms, having more muscle equates to burning more fat. Without engaging in weight training, the risk of losing muscle mass and subsequently compromising metabolic rates looms large. Therefore, neglecting weight lifting could impair both muscle retention and metabolic efficiency, hindering the journey toward fat loss.

The misconception that weightlifting solely burns calories during the workout session is debunked by its significant impact on post-workout metabolism. Weight training triggers a heightened metabolic state for hours post-exercise, facilitating continuous calorie burn even after leaving the gym. Consequently, weightlifting serves as a catalyst for sustained fat burning, extending far beyond the immediate workout period.

Outlined below is a comprehensive fat loss workout program:

Weekly Routine Overview:

Monday: Focus on Chest, Shoulders, and Triceps

Tuesday: Cardio and Abs Training

Wednesday: Emphasis on Quads, Hamstrings, and Calves

Thursday: Cardio and Abs Training

Friday: Concentration on Back, Biceps, and Forearms

Saturday: Rest Day

Sunday: Rest Day

This workout regimen is strategically designed to target different muscle groups across the week, incorporating a blend of weight training and cardiovascular exercises. By following this routine, individuals can expect a comprehensive and intense workout plan that maximizes fat loss potential. The significance of weightlifting as the linchpin of this fat loss program, promising rapid and tangible results.

Furthermore, the emphasis on alternating muscle groups alongside dedicated rest days ensures proper recovery and prevents overtraining, enabling participants to maintain consistency and achieve optimal outcomes.

In conclusion, weight training's crucial role in fat loss cannot be overstated. Integrating weightlifting into a well-structured workout routine not only aids in preserving muscle mass but also contributes significantly to sustained fat burning and metabolic enhancement. Guru Mann's meticulously crafted 10-

week program serves as a testament to the effectiveness of incorporating weight training as a cornerstone of a successful fat loss journey.

Cardiovascular exercise, often referred to as cardio, stands as an indispensable component of any workout regimen. Its significance lies in its unparalleled ability to incinerate fat at an exceptional rate, making it a cornerstone of successful fitness routines. The essence of cardio lies in keeping the body continuously challenged, preventing it from adapting to a singular workout pattern. This constant variation elicits a heightened response from the body, thereby enhancing fat burning and accelerating fitness progress.

The Human Body's Adaptive Nature:

Our bodies possess a remarkable ability to adapt to repetitive workout routines. While consistency in exercise is crucial, a stagnant workout regimen can lead to reduced calorie burn as the body becomes accustomed to the routine. This adaptation results in diminishing returns, impeding the desired results and slowing down progress. Cardio emerges as a dynamic solution to counteract this phenomenon, preventing the body from plateauing and ensuring consistent fat burning.

The Accelerated Fat-Burning Potential of Cardio:

The core benefit of incorporating cardio into workouts lies in its efficacy in torching fat. Engaging in cardio exercises elevates the heart rate and oxygen consumption, prompting the body to utilize stored fat as a primary energy source. This heightened metabolic state during cardio sessions triggers a substantial calorie burn, contributing significantly to overall fat loss.

Variety: The Key to Sustained Progress:

To prevent the body from adapting and plateauing, it's crucial to introduce variety into the workout routine. This diversity can encompass various forms of cardio, such as running, cycling, swimming, or HIIT (High-Intensity Interval Training). These diverse cardio exercises not only challenge different muscle groups but also prevent monotony, thereby keeping the body responsive and consistently burning calories.

Maximizing Cardio's Potential:

For optimal results, consider implementing the following strategies:

Interval Training: Incorporate intervals of high and low intensity within cardio sessions. This approach intensifies calorie burn and spikes the metabolic rate, fostering efficient fat loss.

Cross-Training: Combine different cardio exercises to target multiple muscle groups and prevent boredom. Mix up activities to keep the body adaptable and responsive.

Progressive Overload: Gradually increase the intensity, duration, or frequency of cardio workouts. This method continuously challenges the body, preventing stagnation and ensuring continued fat burning.

Consistency and Persistence: Commitment to a consistent cardio routine is key. Regularity in workouts facilitates habit formation and amplifies the body's response to exercise.

The Road to Results:

Incorporating cardio into a workout routine is not just about shedding fat; it's a strategic approach to optimizing fitness and overall health. By embracing the dynamic nature of cardio exercises and employing diverse techniques, individuals can break through plateaus, maintain consistent fat burn, and expedite progress toward their fitness goals.

Remember, the key lies in keeping the body guessing, adapting, and responding – a principle that underscores the crucial role of cardio in achieving sustained fat loss and overall fitness improvement.

Aerobic exercises stand as a fundamental element within any comprehensive fat loss program. Despite their pivotal role, an effective strategy entails a balanced incorporation of aerobic workouts. Limiting cardio sessions to twice a week, each lasting 30 minutes, presents an optimal approach for initiating significant fat burning while simultaneously stimulating metabolic rates.

Aerobic exercises, commonly known as cardio, serve as an essential tool in the fat loss arsenal due to their ability to trigger substantial fat burning effects. However, the key lies not only in the frequency but also in the strategy and duration of these workouts. Limiting cardio sessions to two sessions weekly is a deliberate approach aimed at leveraging maximum benefits without jeopardizing other crucial aspects of a well-rounded fitness routine.

The Importance of Cardio Frequency:

Aerobic exercises induce a heightened metabolic state that contributes to increased calorie expenditure during and after the workout. Incorporating cardio twice a week allows the body to initiate and sustain fat-burning processes without risking metabolic slowdown. This strategic balance prevents the body from adapting to a routine too quickly, ensuring consistent progress in fat loss goals.

Revving Up the Metabolic Rate:

Contrary to popular belief, excessive cardio sessions might lead to diminishing returns by slowing down the metabolic rate. By restricting aerobic exercises to two sessions per week, each lasting 30 minutes, the body is prompted to respond optimally, revving up the metabolic rate without causing overtraining or potential plateaus.

Adaptation and Monitoring:

Should progress stagnate or individuals find themselves in a rut, the option of increasing cardio sessions to 4-5 times a week may be considered. However, such adjustments must be accompanied by vigilant monitoring of weight room performance and signs of overtraining. The delicate balance between cardiovascular workouts and other aspects of the fitness routine must be maintained to prevent fatigue, decreased performance, or potential injury.

Strategies to Optimize Aerobic Workouts:

To extract the maximum benefits from limited cardio sessions, consider the following strategies:

High-Intensity Interval Training (HIIT): Incorporate HIIT protocols within the 30-minute sessions to amplify calorie burn and metabolic response. Alternating between high-intensity bursts and recovery periods significantly enhances fat loss potential.

Cross-Training: Introduce variety into cardio workouts by integrating different exercises such as cycling, running, swimming, or rowing. This approach targets diverse muscle groups, keeps the body challenged, and prevents monotony.

Monitoring Progress: Track weight room performance, endurance levels, and overall well-being to gauge the impact of aerobic workouts. Any signs of decreased performance or excessive fatigue indicate the need for adjustments in the workout routine.

Prioritize Recovery: Adequate rest and recovery periods between cardio sessions are crucial for muscle repair and overall recovery. Balancing intensity with sufficient rest aids in avoiding overtraining and ensures sustainable progress.

In summary, the strategic incorporation of aerobics, limiting cardio to two sessions weekly lasting 30 minutes each, serves as a catalyst for effective fat loss without compromising metabolic rates or risking overtraining. Monitoring performance indicators and being attentive to the body's responses are key to optimizing aerobic workouts within a comprehensive fitness regimen.

Weight training stands as a critical, yet often overlooked, component in the pursuit of fat loss. Contrary to popular belief, excluding weight training from fitness routines during weight loss endeavors can prove to be a costly mistake. This omission jeopardizes muscle preservation and conditioning, potentially leading to muscle loss as the body resorts to using muscle as an energy source. Muscle loss during dieting presents a significant obstacle, as muscle demands a substantial amount of calories for maintenance. Essentially, the more muscle one possesses, the more effectively fat is burned. Therefore, neglecting weight training undermines muscle retention, consequently impairing the metabolic rate – a dieter's worst nightmare.

The Significance of Muscle Preservation:

In the pursuit of fat loss, it's imperative to understand that weight training plays a pivotal role in preserving muscle mass. When dieting, the body tends to seek energy sources, and without weight training to maintain muscle, it utilizes muscle tissue for fuel. This phenomenon not only sabotages fat loss goals but also undermines metabolic efficiency, as muscle plays a crucial role in sustaining a higher metabolic rate.

Elevated Metabolism Beyond the Weight Room:

Weight lifting's influence extends far beyond the immediate workout session. It induces a metabolic spike that persists for hours post-exercise. This prolonged effect elevates the metabolic rate, resulting in continued calorie burn even after leaving the gym. Thus, weight training becomes a powerful tool in driving fat loss, as it contributes significantly to sustained calorie expenditure throughout the day.

The Backbone of an Effective Fat Loss Program:

A well-structured weight lifting routine forms the cornerstone of an efficient fat loss program. Embracing a fast-paced and vigorous approach to weight training yields equally rapid and impactful results. This regimen not only aids in preserving muscle but also enhances fat burning and metabolic efficiency.

Strategies for Effective Weight Training:

To maximize the benefits of weight training within a fat loss program, consider the following strategies:

Compound Movements: Incorporate compound exercises that engage multiple muscle groups simultaneously. Movements like squats, deadlifts, bench presses, and pull-ups prove highly effective in stimulating muscle growth and overall fat loss.

Progressive Overload: Gradually increase the intensity, resistance, or repetitions in workouts to continuously challenge muscles and stimulate growth. This approach ensures consistent progress and prevents plateauing.

High-Intensity Training: Implement high-intensity interval training (HIIT) techniques within weightlifting sessions. This strategy enhances calorie burn, boosts metabolism, and accelerates fat loss.

Adequate Recovery: Allow sufficient time for muscle recovery between weightlifting sessions. Rest and proper nutrition are vital for muscle repair and growth.

In summary, incorporating weight training into a fat loss regimen is indispensable for preserving muscle mass, elevating metabolic rates, and fostering efficient fat burning. By embracing a dynamic and intense weight lifting routine, individuals can harness its power to sculpt their bodies, promote fat loss, and achieve long-lasting fitness goals.

Chapter 15

EMBARKING ON A WEIGHT loss journey can be challenging, and often individuals encounter stumbling blocks that hinder their progress. Understanding these common pitfalls and implementing quick fixes is essential to stay on track and achieve successful weight loss. Here are some prevalent weight loss traps and effective remedies to overcome them:

Skipping Breakfast:

Trap: Skipping breakfast leads to unhealthy snacking or overeating later in the day.

Fix: Opt for fibre-rich breakfasts like wholegrain bread or porridge to curb mid-morning cravings and stabilize hunger levels.

Skipping Meals:

Trap: Skipping any meal leads to increased hunger and potential overeating later.

Fix: Eat regularly and avoid starving yourself. Keep healthier snacks handy to prevent extreme hunger.

Losing Track of Calories:

Trap: Mindless snacking can disrupt a well-planned diet by increasing calorie intake.

Fix: Keep a food diary to track every bite and stay within your calorie allowance.

Unhealthy Snacking:

Trap: High-calorie snacks contribute to weight gain.

Fix: Choose fibre-rich snacks such as fruits, vegetables, and wholegrain foods to manage hunger and sustain energy levels.

Misconception with 'Low-Fat' Foods:

Trap: 'Low-fat' doesn't always equate to low-calorie.

Fix: Read food labels to check for fat, sugar, and calorie content, not just the fat-free label.

Consuming Calories through Drinks:

Trap: Certain drinks like fancy coffees, sodas, smoothies, and alcoholic beverages are high in calories.

Fix: Opt for low-calorie alternatives like water with lemon, tea or coffee with reduced-fat milk, or herbal tea.

Excessive Weighing:

Trap: Daily weighing may not reflect true weight loss due to natural fluctuations.

Fix: Weigh yourself weekly and rely on other markers of progress like inches lost or how your clothes fit.

Setting Unrealistic Goals:

Trap: Unrealistic weight loss expectations often lead to disappointment.

Fix: Set achievable, smaller goals that contribute to long-term success rather than aiming for drastic weight loss in a short time.

Overeating Post-Exercise:

Trap: Overcompensating for calories burned during exercise can hinder weight loss efforts.

Fix: Opt for low-calorie post-workout snacks and be mindful of portions to avoid undoing the calorie deficit achieved through exercise.

Oversized Portions:

Trap: Large portion sizes contribute to overeating and hinder weight loss.

Fix: Use smaller plates and practice mindful eating, stopping before feeling full to control portion sizes.

By being aware of these common weight loss pitfalls and implementing these practical fixes, individuals can navigate their weight loss journey more effectively. Making small, sustainable changes and being mindful of dietary habits and portions are key to achieving successful and lasting weight loss results.

In an ideal scenario, the support of family and friends would seamlessly align with your weekly weight loss endeavor. However, the reality often presents challenges as loved ones inadvertently contribute to peer pressure, leading to deviations from your goals. Whether it's a friend tempting you with "just one more drink" or a partner suggesting to skip the gym for dinner, these well-meaning encouragements can derail your progress. To resist peer pressure and stay on track with your daily calorie allowance, consider the following strategies:

Seek Home Support:

Communicate the importance of their support to your family. Engaging them in your journey can make them more sensitive to your goals and struggles.

Request Temptation-Free Environment:

Ask those around you not to offer your favorite treats to avoid succumbing to temptation. Creating an environment that supports your choices is crucial.

Pre-plan Social Events:

Plan ahead for evenings out by adjusting your calorie intake earlier in the day. This strategy ensures you stay within your daily allowance despite social outings.

Avoid Drinking Rounds:

Steer clear of rounds at the pub that might pressure you to match your friends' drinking pace. Opt to buy your own drinks to maintain control over your consumption.

Pre-Decide Meals When Eating Out:

Review restaurant menus online before dining out and decide on your meal in advance. Having a plan in place helps you make healthier choices.

Practice Assertiveness:

Learn to politely decline unwanted food or drinks offered by loved ones. Saying no firmly but courteously reinforces your commitment without being rude.

Celebrate Milestones:

Share your achievements with your support network. Letting them know when you reach milestones reinforces your dedication and helps them understand the significance of your goals.

Navigating peer pressure during your weight loss journey requires a delicate balance between asserting your goals and maintaining healthy relationships. By involving loved ones, setting boundaries, and pre-planning for social situations, you can stay aligned with your objectives while nurturing supportive connections. Remember, staying committed to your goals and communicating your progress effectively helps build understanding and encouragement within your social circle.

When striving to adopt healthier habits and manage food temptations, engaging in various activities with friends proves to be an effective way to shift focus from food-centric gatherings. Here's a compilation of enjoyable and diverting pursuits that can help you spend quality time with friends while steering clear of food-centric situations:

Country Walks:

Embrace nature's beauty by taking serene strolls in the countryside. These walks not only provide a peaceful escape but also offer a chance for meaningful conversations amidst the tranquil surroundings.

Cinema Escapades with Homemade Low-Calorie Popcorn:

Enjoy an evening at the movies while bringing your own low-calorie popcorn. This way, you indulge in a snack without sacrificing your dietary goals.

Bowling Fun:

Unleash your competitive spirit and bond with friends over a game of bowling. The physical activity involved adds an element of exercise to the entertainment.

Bike Rides and Picnics (with Low-Calorie Delights):

Embark on a bike ride and complement it with a thoughtfully prepared, low-calorie picnic. Delight in the outdoor setting while relishing healthier snack options.

Roller-Skating Adventures:

Experience the thrill of roller-skating while spending quality time with friends. It's a fantastic way to exercise and engage in laughter-filled moments.

Playful Sports:

Enjoy a game of Frisbee or football at the park. Not only does it foster camaraderie, but it also promotes physical activity and a sense of team spirit.

Engaging in these diverse activities not only offers an opportunity to bond with friends but also helps divert attention away from food-centric socializing. They provide avenues for physical activity, laughter, and shared experiences that contribute to overall well-being without the emphasis on food. Prioritizing such activities not only supports your health goals but also strengthens friendships through shared moments of joy and fun.

Navigating weight loss goals while dining out is a considerable challenge for many individuals embarking on a healthier lifestyle. The allure of diverse menu options coupled with social pressures often complicates efforts to adhere to dietary objectives during restaurant visits. Temptations abound, enticing diners with indulgent, high-calorie dishes that might derail their weight loss journey. Making healthier choices amidst such culinary temptations demands strategy, mindfulness, and a proactive approach.

The restaurant environment, with its array of delectable dishes, poses a significant temptation for individuals striving to adhere to healthier eating habits. The tantalizing descriptions and visually appealing presentations of calorie-laden meals often test one's resolve. Managing portion sizes and resisting the appeal of rich, flavorful options can be overwhelming, particularly when surrounded by friends or family who indulge in such choices.

Identifying and choosing healthier options from restaurant menus isn't always straightforward. The healthier selections may lack prominence or fail to captivate attention compared to the more decadent offerings. Additionally, dining out is often associated with larger portion sizes, making it challenging to practice moderation and adhere to recommended calorie intake.

Social dynamics play a pivotal role in dining-out experiences, further complicating weight loss efforts. Peer pressure and the desire to conform to social norms might lead individuals to deviate from their intended dietary path. The fear of being perceived as overly restrictive or unsociable often nudges individuals toward indulging in high-calorie meals or consuming larger portions than planned.

Successfully navigating these challenges involves adopting proactive strategies and mindful decision-making. Pre-planning by reviewing restaurant menus in advance helps in identifying healthier options and planning meals to align with dietary goals. Opting for dishes featuring lean proteins, vegetables, or whole grains and requesting modifications can contribute to healthier meal choices.

Portion control is vital; individuals can consider sharing meals or packing leftovers to manage portion sizes and prevent overeating. Choosing beverages wisely, such as opting for water or unsweetened options, helps curb additional calorie intake. Communicating dietary preferences to friends or dining companions beforehand fosters understanding and support, minimizing social pressure.

When faced with indulgent menu choices, strategies like sharing appetizers or splitting desserts among friends allow individuals to enjoy the flavors without overindulging. Balancing indulgent meals with lighter options in subsequent meals helps maintain overall calorie balance. Embracing mindful eating practices, fostering gratitude, and understanding the occasional need for flexibility contribute to a positive dining experience while aligning with weight loss goals.

In conclusion, navigating weight loss aspirations while dining out necessitates a mindful, balanced approach. Overcoming the allure of indulgent dishes, managing portion sizes, and negotiating social influences requires proactive decision-making. By integrating pre-planning, mindful choices, and balanced eating practices, individuals can savor dining experiences without compromising their commitment to healthier lifestyles.

Chapter 16

DINING OUT IS A DELIGHTFUL experience, but it can challenge our commitment to healthier eating habits. Fear not! Navigating menus while keeping calorie counts in check doesn't have to be a daunting task. With some thoughtful strategies, you can relish the occasion without jeopardizing your dietary goals.

Strategic Menu Reconnaissance:

Before stepping into the restaurant, take advantage of technology. Checking the restaurant's menu online grants you a tactical advantage. It allows for preemptive planning, identifying lower-calorie options, and estimating your expected calorie intake. Armed with this information, making informed, healthier choices becomes more manageable and lessens the pull of temptation.

Consistency in Meal Timing:

Skipping meals as a form of calorie accumulation for an evening out is counterproductive. Maintain your daily meal routine, including breakfast and lunch, to regulate appetite throughout the day. Should you exceed your calorie allowance during the dining experience, simply recalibrate by reducing intake in the subsequent days to maintain balance.

Portion Moderation:

One course is perfectly acceptable. No need to feel obligated to consume multiple courses. Practice portion control; halt eating before feeling overly full. Opting for a starter or side dish as your main course can curb the tendency to overeat.

Mindful Selection of Preparations:

Steering clear of deep-fried or battered dishes is advisable, as these preparations tend to be high in fat content. Opt for grilled, roasted, steamed, or baked options. Avoid sauces laden with cheese, cream, or butter, opting instead for tomato-based or vegetable sauces that are lower in fat content.

Navigating Salads and Dressings:

Exercise caution with salads as they may harbor high-calorie toppings such as cheese, bacon, nuts, or croutons. Request salad dressing on the side to control the amount added, ensuring you only incorporate as much as necessary.

Savor the Experience:

Eating slowly and relishing each bite is key. This method not only induces satisfaction before feeling overly full but also offers more opportunities to engage in conversation and absorb the ambiance.

Dessert Strategy:

Opt for healthier dessert choices like fruit-based options or crumbles. Should the allure of a decadent dessert prove irresistible, consider sharing it with a companion to savor the taste without consuming the entire portion.

Beverage Consciousness:

Be wary of liquid calories, especially in alcoholic beverages and sugary soft drinks. Choosing water or sugar-free alternatives over high-calorie options can significantly contribute to managing overall caloric intake.

By implementing these strategies while dining out, you can maintain a balance between relishing delicious meals and adhering to your calorie goals. Planning ahead, practicing moderation, and making mindful selections empower you to enjoy dining experiences while staying on track with your dietary aspirations.

Exploring international cuisine is an exciting journey filled with diverse flavors. However, when aiming to opt for healthier choices within these culinary adventures, specific considerations can help navigate menus to choose lower-calorie options.

Italian Delicacies:

When savoring Italian fare, exercising caution with cheese and cream-based pasta sauces like alfredo or carbonara can significantly impact calorie intake. Opt for thin-crust pizzas topped with vegetables, tomato-based sauces, vegetable-based soups, or grilled dishes for a lighter indulgence. Steer clear of indulgences like cheesy or meaty pizzas, salami, creamy sauces, garlic bread, or lasagne that are higher in calories.

Chinese Cuisine:

Navigating Chinese cuisine can be rewarding when avoiding sweet sauces and fried dishes. Opt for healthier alternatives like stir-fries, steamed dumplings, vegetables, plain boiled rice, and steamed fish or chicken. Be cautious of high-calorie choices such as deep-fried options, sweet and sour dishes, prawn toast, spring rolls, or egg fried rice that tend to be richer in calories.

Thai Temptations:

Thai cuisine offers ample opportunities for healthier choices, often featuring steamed or stir-fried vegetables. Opt for salads, stir-fries, steamed rice, and broth-based soups for lower-calorie options. However, avoid coconut milk-based dishes, fried rice, peanut sauce, or crispy noodles that tend to pack more calories.

Indian Varieties:

Despite the reliance on frying in some Indian dishes, numerous healthier choices exist. Opt for tomato-based sauces, tandoori dishes, or plain/basmati rice for lower-calorie options. Be wary of calorie-dense items such as bhajis, poppadoms, creamy curries, pilau rice, or naan bread.

By selectively opting for these lower-calorie choices while exploring foreign cuisines, one can relish the diverse flavors without compromising dietary goals. Making mindful selections that emphasize steamed, grilled, or stir-fried options over cream-based, deep-fried, or calorie-dense dishes allows for a more balanced culinary experience.

Chapter 17

HARNESSING THE POWER of Fruits and Vegetables for Weight Management:

Incorporating a diverse range of fruits and vegetables into our daily diet is not just a health recommendation; it's a beneficial strategy for weight management too. These natural wonders are rich in fiber, vitamins, and minerals while being low in calories, making them an ideal addition to a balanced diet. The fiber content aids in digestion, provides a feeling of fullness, and helps regulate blood sugar levels, contributing to weight management goals. Nutritionists often advocate for consuming at least five portions of various fruits and vegetables daily to reap their numerous health benefits while assisting in weight management.

Deceptive Salads and Their Caloric Traps:

While salads are frequently touted as a go-to for health-conscious individuals and those striving to manage their weight, not all salads are created equal. Beneath the veil of fresh greens and colorful vegetables, several hidden factors might compromise the healthfulness of these seemingly virtuous meals. Condiments, dressings, toppings, and add-ons can substantially elevate the calorie count of a salad, potentially sabotaging your weight management efforts.

Navigating Salad Pitfalls:

Dressings and Sauces: Creamy dressings or heavy vinaigrettes can add excess calories. Opt for lighter alternatives like balsamic vinaigrette or request dressings on the side to control portions.

Toppings and Add-ons: Ingredients like cheese, bacon bits, croutons, candied nuts, or dried fruits contribute to increased calorie content. Exercise caution with these toppings or opt for smaller quantities or healthier alternatives.

Protein Choices: While proteins like grilled chicken or tofu are healthy additions, they might be prepared with high-calorie marinades or coatings. Choose lean proteins and inquire about preparation methods to avoid hidden fats.

Portion Size: Salad portions served at restaurants or pre-packaged salads can sometimes exceed recommended sizes. Be mindful of portion sizes and, if possible, split larger portions or take some home for later.

Hidden Sugar and Sodium: Salad dressings, particularly pre-made or bottled ones, may contain added sugars or high sodium content. Reading labels and opting for homemade or low-sugar alternatives can be beneficial.

Crafting Healthier Salads:

To make salads more weight-management friendly, focus on loading up on fresh leafy greens and a variety of colorful vegetables. Opt for lean proteins, portion control, homemade dressings using healthier ingredients, and limit high-calorie toppings or add-ons. Preparing salads at home allows for better control over ingredients and portion sizes, ensuring a healthier and more weight-conscious meal.

In summary, while fruits, vegetables, and salads are excellent dietary components, exercising caution with salad ingredients, dressings, and portion sizes can impact their healthfulness. By making informed choices, monitoring portions, and opting for healthier alternatives, salads can remain a valuable asset in a weight management plan without compromising health goals.

Harnessing the Power of Vegetables in Evening Meals:

Incorporating vegetables into evening meals is a fantastic strategy to elevate nutritional intake and support weight management goals. Committing to including at least two portions of vegetables in every evening meal presents a golden opportunity to boost fiber, vitamins, and minerals in your diet. Whether steamed, roasted, stir-fried, or incorporated into main dishes, vegetables offer a variety of flavors and textures to enhance the dining experience while promoting health and wellness.

Exploring Homemade Salads and Culinary Creativity:

Experimenting with homemade salads provides an excellent avenue for culinary exploration and healthier eating habits. Get creative with colorful greens, an assortment of vegetables, fruits, nuts, seeds, lean proteins, and dressings to craft nutritious and flavorful salads. Incorporating diverse ingredients not only enriches the nutritional profile but also adds excitement to meals, making salads a delightful and satisfying option for lunch or dinner.

Prioritizing Lunchtime Walks for Physical Activity:

Allocating time for three 30-minute lunchtime walks during the week presents an opportune moment to infuse physical activity into daily routines. Your lunch break can be transformed into an active period, offering a refreshing break from sedentary tasks. Whether a brisk walk outdoors or a stroll in a nearby park, these walks not only contribute to burning calories but also help in reducing stress, boosting mood, and enhancing overall well-being.

Commitment to Calorie and Exercise Targets:

Sticking to predetermined calorie intake and exercise goals forms the bedrock of successful weight management endeavors. Consistency in monitoring and maintaining the balance between calorie consumption and physical activity aids in achieving and sustaining weight-related objectives. Whether through meal planning, portion control, regular exercise routines, or tracking progress, adherence to these targets significantly contributes to a healthier lifestyle.

In essence, these strategies encompass a holistic approach to a healthier lifestyle. By consciously integrating more vegetables into meals, experimenting with homemade salads, incorporating lunchtime walks, and staying committed to calorie and exercise targets, individuals can cultivate habits that promote health, wellness, and sustainable weight management. These small, manageable steps contribute significantly to long-term well-being and a balanced lifestyle.

Enhancing Weight Loss Efforts with Vegetables:

Integrating a higher intake of vegetables into your daily meals is a potent strategy for aiding weight loss and maintaining a healthier lifestyle. Vegetables, rich in fiber, vitamins, and minerals, play a crucial role in weight management. Their high fiber content not only contributes to satiety but also offers a low-calorie density, making them an ideal component of a weight loss diet.

The Role of Vegetables in Weight Loss:

Vegetables possess a unique quality due to their fiber content that helps in providing a feeling of fullness without significantly increasing calorie intake. By incorporating a variety of vegetables into your meals, you can enjoy satisfying and wholesome dishes while staying within your daily calorie allowance. This approach helps curb hunger pangs between meals, contributing to better control over calorie consumption.

Ten Tips to Incorporate More Vegetables:

Meal Filling with Vegetables: Increase the volume of your meals by adding vegetables while reducing higher-calorie ingredients or portion sizes, facilitating a feeling of fullness with fewer calories.

Legumes and Pulses: Introduce beans, lentils, and pulses into stews, salads, and bakes to enhance both nutritional value and satiety.

Diverse Vegetable Portions: Aim for at least two portions of vegetables on your plate, whether it's peas with shepherd's pie or carrots and broccoli in a roast dinner.

Vegetable-Based Dishes: Incorporate more salads or vegetable-centric meals that can provide multiple servings of your recommended daily vegetable intake while offering a variety of flavors and textures.

Vegetable Snacks: Opt for convenient and easy-to-pack vegetable snacks like baby carrots, radishes, or sugar snap peas to satisfy hunger between meals.

Sauce Swaps: Substitute cheese or cream-based sauces with tomato or vegetable-based alternatives, enhancing the nutritional profile of your meals and making them more filling.

Sandwich Enhancements: Amp up the nutritional content of your sandwiches by adding vegetables like lettuce, tomatoes, cucumbers, or grated carrots for added crunch and satiety.

Frozen Vegetable Convenience: Utilize frozen vegetables as a quick and hassle-free option for meal preparation, providing a range of choices from single vegetables to mixed varieties.

Healthier Breakfast Options: Opt for healthier breakfast choices by swapping fried options with grilled vegetables like tomatoes or mushrooms or incorporating onions and peppers into omelettes.

Leafy Greens in Meals: Incorporate calcium and iron-rich leafy greens such as kale or Swiss chard into soups or stews, elevating both taste and nutritional value effortlessly.

By adopting these ten tips and incorporating a diverse range of vegetables into your meals, you can not only enhance your weight loss journey but also enrich your diet with vital nutrients essential for overall well-being.

Unlocking the Potential of Salads in Weight Loss:

Salads serve as an ally in weight loss journeys, offering a nutrient-dense and low-calorie option for satiating hunger. However, caution is warranted against calorie-dense toppings that can potentially sabotage your weight loss efforts. A basic green salad comprising fresh greens, tomatoes, and cucumbers is low in calories, salt, and fat, while rich in essential nutrients.

Navigating the Salad Minefield:

Despite the healthful core ingredients, the potential calorie bomb in salads lies in the toppings. Croutons, bacon bits, cheese, breaded chicken, and creamy dressings can transform an otherwise healthy salad into a calorie-loaded meal. To maintain the integrity of a weight-conscious salad, the rule of thumb is to steer clear of fatty toppings, request dressings on the side, and opt out of mayonnaise or cream-based dressings.

The Dressing Dilemma:

Salad dressings, while enhancing taste, often pack a calorie punch. A mere two tablespoons of mayonnaise can add 220kcal to your meal, while mayo-based Thousand Island dressing contributes 194kcal, and blue cheese dressing boasts 228kcal.

Strategies for Healthier Dressings:

Crafting lower-fat, lower-calorie dressings using fruit juices or opting for healthier alternatives like olive oil and vinegar or fresh lemon juice can significantly reduce calorie intake.

Caution is advised with commercial lower-fat salad dressings as they may compensate for reduced fat content with increased sugar. Always scrutinize the nutrition label for hidden sugars.

When dining out, request that dressings be served on the side, allowing you to add only as much as necessary, exercising control over calorie intake.

Certain salads like Caesar, Waldorf, coleslaw, and some pasta and potato variations tend to be drenched in mayonnaise, thereby packing excess calories. It's advisable to approach these cautiously or seek healthier alternatives.

By exercising vigilance and opting for nutrient-rich salad components while steering clear of calorie-laden toppings and dressings, salads can become a cornerstone of your weight loss regime. Smart choices in salad ingredients and dressings empower you to enjoy a flavorful and satisfying meal that aligns with your weight management goals.

Chapter 18

OVERCOMING WEIGHT LOSS Setbacks:

Encountering setbacks is a common part of any weight loss journey. How you respond to these challenges defines your ultimate success. Here are practical fixes for some common obstacles:

1. Expecting Setbacks:

It's normal to yield to temptation occasionally. If you slip up and indulge in something outside your plan, don't let it derail your progress. Acknowledge the slip, let it go, and refocus immediately. One moment of indulgence shouldn't overshadow your entire journey.

2. Managing Hunger Pangs:

Persistent hunger doesn't have to be a part of your weight loss efforts. Ensure you're adhering to your daily calorie limit without undercutting it drastically. Incorporate fiber-rich, low-calorie foods into your diet to keep hunger at bay while feeling fuller for longer.

3. Staying Motivated:

Weight loss endeavors can be demanding. Set mini-goals throughout your journey, rewarding yourself when achieved. These goals need not be solely about weight; they can be behavioral or lifestyle-related milestones. Celebrate your victories with non-food rewards to keep motivation high.

4. Patience with Inches vs. Weight Loss:

Body fat distribution varies, impacting how and where weight is lost. Initially, weight loss might precede visible inch reduction. Patience is key; with time, you'll notice changes as your body adjusts, clothes start fitting differently, and your physique becomes leaner.

5. Overcoming Plateaus:

Weight loss plateaus are common. Ensure strict adherence to your calorie limit, scrutinize portion sizes, and be vigilant about snacks. To break through plateaus, consider tweaking your exercise routine, introducing new challenges for your body, or increasing physical activity.

By embracing setbacks as part of the journey and responding with resilience, mindfulness, and adaptability, you'll navigate these obstacles more effectively, propelling yourself closer to your weight loss goals.

Make your own workout plan here.

Don't miss out!

Click the button below and you can sign up to receive emails whenever Jagdish Krishanlal Arora publishes a new book. There's no charge and no obligation.

Did you love *How to Lose Weight Quickly*? Then you should read <u>*Mental Health and Well Being*</u> by Jagdish Krishanlal Arora!

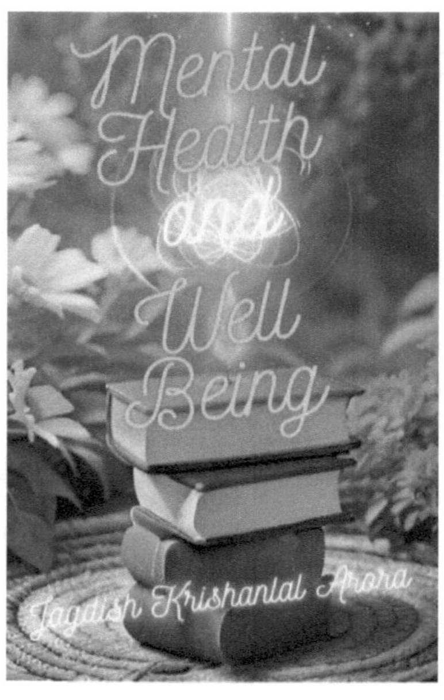

In the fast-paced and often turbulent world we live in, the significance of mental health and well-being has never been more profound. This book is an exploration into the depths of our emotional and psychological landscapes, a journey that traverses the intricacies of the human mind and soul. It is an invitation to embark on a transformative quest towards understanding, nurturing, and enhancing the most vital aspect of our existence – our mental well-being.

As we go into the pages of this book, we will uncover a tapestry of stories, insights, and practical exercises that illuminate the path to mental health and well-being. From mindfulness practices that ground us in the present moment to exercises in resilience-building that empower us to face life's challenges, this book offers a comprehensive guide to enriching our inner world. Whether you're seeking solace from emotional turmoil, striving for personal growth, or simply curious about the intricacies of the human mind, this book is a beacon of wisdom and compassion on the journey to lasting well-being.

Also by Jagdish Krishanlal Arora

Basic Inorganic and Organic Chemistry
Book of Jokes
Car Insurance and Claims
Digital Electronics, Computer Architecture and
Microprocessor Design Principles
Guided Meditation and Yoga
The Bible and Jesus Christ
Unity Quest
From Oasis to Global Stage: The Evolution of Arab
Civilization
Secrets of Mount Kailash, Bermuda Triangle and the
Lost City of Atlantis
Visitors from Outer Space
Motivation
The Aliens and God Theory
The Lunar Voyager
Queen Elizabeth II and the British Monarchy
The Kremlin Conspiracy
Vegetable Gardening, Salads and Recipes
How to End The War in Ukraine
The Old and New World Order
Travelling to Mars in the Cosmic Odyssey 2050
Romance Pays Off
How the Universe Works
Mental Health and Well Being
Ancient History of Mars
The Nexus
Basic and Advanced Physics

Administrative Law
Calculus
The Ramayana
A Watery Mystery
Romantic Conflicts
Thieves of Palestine
Love in Chicago
WordPress Design and Development
Travellers Guide to Mount Kailash
Become a Better Writer With Creative Writing
Emerging Trends in Carbon Emission Reduction
India Independence Through Non Violence
Copyright, Patents, Trademarks and Trade Secret
Laws
Decoding CHATGPT and Artificial Intelligence
The Untold Story of Diana and Prince Charles
Time Travel
How to Lose Weight Quickly

www.ingramcontent.com/pod-product-compliance
Lightning Source LLC
Chambersburg PA
CBHW031402250726
48656CB00002B/533